Studying the Organisation and Delivery of Health Services

There is increasing recognition that advances in medicine are only part of the answer to better health care. These advances, together with rising expectations of health care users, mean that demands on the way we organise and deliver services will become even greater. It is therefore essential that we advance our understanding and knowledge of how best to organise and deliver health services. This book, written by experienced teachers and researchers, introduces research methods from a wide range of disciplines and applies them to research on the organisation and delivery of health services.

Each chapter takes a different discipline or approach and provides: a definition and description of its theoretical basis; advice on and examples of the types of research question it can appropriately address; a description of its methods – their uses and limitations; a list of further reading.

Disciplines and approaches covered include: epidemiology; sociology; organisational psychology; action research; organisational studies; political science/policy analysis; economics; historical methods and operational research. The book also looks at the issues in synthesising evidence from qualitative research and non-experimental quantitative studies.

This is an invaluable reader for researchers, students and research funders and provides an appropriate text for the growing number of courses in the multidisciplinary field of health services research.

Naomi Fulop is Senior Lecturer in Health Service Delivery and Organisational Research, **Pauline Allen** is Lecturer in Organisational Research, **Aileen Clarke** is Senior Lecturer in Public Health and **Nick Black** is Professor of Health Services Research; all are from the London School of Hygiene and Tropical Medicine and are involved in the centre supporting the new NHS research and development programme in Health Service Delivery and Organisation.

Studying the Organisation and Delivery of Health Services

Research methods

Edited by Naomi Fulop,
Pauline Allen, Aileen Clarke
and Nick Black

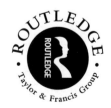

London and New York

First published 2001
by Routledge
11 New Fetter Lane, London EC4P 4EE

Simultaneously published in the USA and Canada
by Routledge
29 West 35th Street, New York, NY 10001

Reprinted 2002

Routledge is an imprint of the Taylor & Francis Group

Typeset in Times by Taylor & Francis Books Ltd

Printed and bound in Great Britain by Biddles Ltd,
Guildford and King's Lynn

British Library Cataloguing in Publication Data
A catalogue record for this book is available from the British
Library

Library of Congress Cataloging in Publication Data
Studying the organisation and delivery of health services :
research methods / edited by Naomi Fulop ... [et al.]
p. cm.
Includes bibliographical references and index.
1. Health services administration–Research–Methodology.
2. Medical care–Research–Methodology.
I. Fulop, Naomi. [DNLM: 1. Delivery of Health Care–
organization & administration. 2. Research–methods.
W 84.1 S933 2001]
RA440.85 .S78 2001
362.1~068–dc21   2001019651

ISBN 0–415–25762–X (hbk)
ISBN 0–415–25763–8 (pbk)

Contents

Illustrations

Figures

Tables

Contributors

Pauline Allen is a lecturer in Organisational Research at the London School of Hygiene and Tropical Medicine and a member of the National Co-ordinating Centre for NHS Service Delivery and Organisation R&D Programme. She is also qualified as a solicitor, although she no longer practises. Using economic and legal approaches, her research interests include contracts, looking at both formal and informal relationships and professional and legal accountability.

John Arnold is Professor of Organisation Behaviour at Loughborough University Business School. His current research interests include career management, work-role transitions, the transition from education to work, psychological contracts at work, managing career development in organisations, commitment and socialisation at work and lifespan development.

Virginia Berridge is Professor of History at the London School of Hygiene and Tropical Medicine. Her research interests include science–policy relationships, twentieth-century health policy, illicit drugs, HIV/AIDS, smoking, alcohol, and the role of the media.

Nick Black is Professor of Health Services Research and Head of Department of Public Health and Policy at the London School of Hygiene and Tropical Medicine. His main interests include quality improvement (particularly in surgery), the relationship between research and policy/practice, and the uses of high-quality clinical databases.

Marion K. Campbell is the Programme Director of Health Care Assessment at the Health Services Research Unit, University of Aberdeen. She directs a programme of research aimed at evaluating new health technologies. Her interest is in clinical trials methodology, particularly the design and statistical analysis of cluster randomised trials.

Aileen Clarke is the Senior Lecturer in Public Health at the London School of Hygiene and Tropical Medicine. Her research interests include health services research, particularly the uptake and dissemination of research evidence, clinical decisions, the decision-making process and the provision of information and decision aids for patients. She is also interested in the use of routine data, for example, readmission to hospital or length of stay to assess the quality of health care.

Diane Dawson is Senior Research Fellow at the Centre for Health Economics, University of York. Her research interests focus on the microeconomics of health care organisation and the impact of regulation. Topics have included the pricing of hospital services, the role of longer-term contracts, and lessons for regulation of health care from other sectors.

Martin P. Eccles is Professor of Clinical Effectiveness at the Centre for Health Services Research at the School of Health Sciences, University of Newcastle upon Tyne. His research interests are in implementation research and methods of guideline development.

Ewan Ferlie is Professor of Public Services Management at Imperial College Management School. His research interests include: the organisation and management of health care services; patterns of organisational change; professional and managerial roles and relationships; new organisational forms; corporate and clinical governance.

Naomi Fulop is Senior Lecturer in Health Service Delivery and Organisational Research and Director of the National Co-ordinating Centre for NHS Service Delivery and Organisation R&D Programme at the London School of Hygiene and Tropical Medicine. Her research interests are in the organisation and management of health care: implementation of health policies; relationships between organisations (mergers, integration, partnerships); and the relationship between research and policy.

Jeremy M. Grimshaw is Programme Director and Professor of Health Services Research at the University of Aberdeen. He conducts a programme of implementation research involving systematic reviews and rigorous evaluations of implementation strategies, and methodological work to test the applicability of psychological models to professional behaviour change and to address design and statistical issues in implementation research.

Steve Harrison is Professor of Social Policy at the University of Manchester. His research interests include health policy and politics, health service organisation, medical/managerial relationships, and user/public involvement. He has a special interest in the politics of 'evidence'.

Nicholas Mays is Advisor, Social Policy Branch, The Treasury, Wellington, New Zealand, and Visiting Professor, Department of Public Health and Policy at the London School of Hygiene and Tropical Medicine. He is a health services researcher and health policy analyst with a particular interest in health systems, the use of quasi-markets in health care, the role of primary care and the impact of organisational change on health services performance.

Julienne Meyer is Professor of Nursing (Care for Older People) at City University St Bartholomew School of Nursing and Midwifery. Her research interests predominantly focus on care for older people, together with user and carer involvement, interprofessional working, and practice development through action research. Much of her work focuses on change and trying to improve the delivery and organisation of health and social care. A key feature, within this, is exploring the value and contribution of nursing within the multidisciplinary team.

Elizabeth Murphy is Reader in Sociology and Social Policy at the University of Nottingham. Her major research interests are in medical sociology, the sociology of food and eating, and the application of qualitative methods to health-related research.

Jennie Popay is Professor of Sociology and Health Policy, Nuffield Institute for Health at the University of Leeds. She has extensive experience of research in the public health field, and has a particular interest in the contribution qualitative research has to make to the understanding of social inequalities in health and to the evidence base for policy and practice in public health. She is coordinator of the Cochrane Qualitative Methods Research Network and convenor of the Campbell Collaboration's Process Evaluation/Diverse Study Designs Methods Group.

Craig R. Ramsay is Senior Statistician at the University of Aberdeen. He conducts a programme of work to address design and statistical issues in implementation research. His interests include quasi-experimental designs, cluster trials and learning-curve effects.

Emilie Roberts is Research Officer, Community Care Programme at the King's Fund. She joined the King's Fund to specialise in literature reviewing, publishing work on emergency care. More recently, she has focused on the health care of older people using a range of research methods. She is currently reviewing the literature on inter-generational equity in UK health policy and service delivery.

Jonathan Rosenhead is Professor of Operational Research at the London School of Economics. His research concerns model-based analysis relevant to problems and issues in health service delivery. This includes, but is not limited to, applications to Accident and Emergency, medical audit, facility location, regional planning and children's health services. His methodological focus is on problem structuring methods, which provide participatory decision support in workshop situations.

Mark Sculpher is Senior Research Fellow at the University of York. His research interests include: the economic evaluation of health care programmes and interventions; methods research in the area of decision modelling and Bayesian approaches to economic evaluation; the implications of shared decision making for health care systems; and benefit valuation in health care.

Brenda Wilson is Senior Lecturer in Public Health/Honorary Consultant in Public Health Medicine at the University of Aberdeen. Her research interests lie in identifying effective and appropriate strategies for preventing cancer and organising cancer services. She also runs a programme of research in post-genome health services, including evaluating different models of service delivery, improving primary care aspects of genetic counselling, and using rigorous techniques to elicit user preferences.

Acknowledgements

We would like to thank the NHS Methodology R&D programme for funding the workshop held in May 2000, where earlier drafts of the chapters were discussed, and the participants for their contributions: Nicky Britten, Stirling Bryan, Martin Buxton, Bronwyn Croxson, Maureen Dalziel, John Gabbay, Alan Glanz, Tony Harrison, David J. Hunter, Richard Lilford, Lorna McKee, John Pattison, Anne Marie Rafferty, Sally Redfern, Colin Sanderson and Jan van der Meulen. We are grateful to Simon Carter for his comments on an earlier version of Chapter 1. We would also like to thank Melanie Ferrier, Margaret Mellor and Linda Philip for their support in the preparation of the manuscript.

The authors of Chapter 4 are funded by the Chief Scientist Office, Scottish Executive Department of Health, and their views are not necessarily held by the funding body. Jonathan Rosenhead (Chapter 10) gratefully acknowledges advice and information received from Gwyn Bevan, Paul Forte, Penny Mullen, Diane Plamping, Geoff Royston and Peter Smith. Nicholas Mays and Emilie Roberts (Chapter 12) acknowledge that their contribution builds on a series of systematic literature reviews of health service organisational and financial interventions undertaken as part of a wider research project funded by the NHS Executive London R&D Programme.

We thank Elsevier Science for permission to reproduce Box 12.8 from Robert and Mays 1998.

We thank Harvard University Press for permission to reproduce Box 12.1 from Light and Pillemer 1984.

We thank the NHS Centre for Reviews and Dissemination (University of York) for permission to reproduce Box 12.2 from CRD Report 4 1996.

We thank Open University Press for permission to reproduce Table 11.1 from Hart and Bond 1995.

We thank the Royal Society of Medicine Press Ltd for permission to reproduce Box 12.5 from Steiner and Robinson 1998.

Three of us (Naomi Fulop, Pauline Allen and Aileen Clarke) are funded by the NHS Service Delivery and Organisation R&D programme. The programme also funded the administrative support provided to produce this book.

Naomi Fulop, Pauline Allen, Aileen Clarke, Nick Black
June 2001

Chapter 1

Issues in studying the organisation and delivery of health services

Naomi Fulop, Pauline Allen, Aileen Clarke and Nick Black

Why study the organisation and delivery of health services?

Throughout the world, societies are striving to determine how best to organise their health systems and deliver services. Increasingly, there is a recognition that the development and evaluation of new therapies and diagnostic tools is only part of the answer to better health care. As we enter a new era of biological understanding of disease following the mapping of the human genome, the demands on the way we organise services will become even greater. This pressure will be enhanced by the rising expectations of consumers and greater access to information. It is essential, therefore, that in parallel to biomedical research and health technology assessment, we advance our understanding and knowledge of how best to organise and deliver health services. Without this, we run the risk of failing to realise the potential benefits that health systems can provide.

In addition, the need to be more responsive to the needs and wishes of those who use health care is increasingly being accepted. The traditional tendency for service organisations to prioritise staff needs over consumers' needs is no longer acceptable, regardless of whether the system is publicly or privately financed.

All of these pressures have led governments to recognise the need to increase their support for research that can help to improve the way we organise and deliver health services. While this is not a new area of study, the previously disjointed, *ad hoc* activities that characterised such research are giving way to a more strategic approach, with national programmes of research in some countries. This, in turn, will require a growth in both the volume and quality of research. To achieve these, the tendency for fragmentation between the very disciplines that can make key contributions must be overcome.

The aim of this book is to go some way towards meeting these challenges. It is aimed at researchers and research funders in the field of health services delivery and organisation who need to be familiar with the range of methods required. They may be experts in one particular field but need to have a working knowledge of how other methods can contribute. Alternatively, they may be new to this field of enquiry. Given the necessity for multidisciplinary working in this area, it is important that researchers and funders are aware of the range of appropriate methods and the types of questions which different methods can address; and further, they need to understand that different methods will generate different insights in the light of the theoretical perspective of the relevant discipline.

A further aim of this book is to explore the extent to which multidisciplinary working can be achieved – whether some disciplines can work together, or whether some disciplines are inherently incompatible. Although we cover a wide range of disciplines and methods, it is not comprehensive – by necessity we have not been able to cover all those which may appropriately be used (for example, anthropology and geography have not been included).

The last two decades have been termed the Era of Assessment and Accountability by Arnold Relman, ex-editor of the *New England Journal of Medicine* (Relman 1998). They were marked by the adoption of scientific management, health technology assessment and the acceptance of evidence-based medicine based on clinical guidelines. While all these developments have contributed to maintaining a working relationship between funders, providers and the public, it is clear that the pressure on health systems persists and is likely to increase. It is time to enter the next era of health care, one in which we attend to the way we organise and deliver services, with much greater involvement of the public and consumers: an era of research on service delivery and organisation (SDO).

In this chapter, first we outline the development of research on the delivery and organisation of health services. Second, we discuss what we call some 'fundamentals': these are the key terms and debates concerning researchers generally, and applying to research in this field. These include matters of epistemology (theory of knowledge), and the relationship between disciplines and methods. Third, we present a brief description of each chapter. Finally, we use an example of an issue in health service delivery and organisation (how best to deliver orthopaedic care) to illustrate how the different disciplines and approaches can be applied.

The development of health service delivery and organisation research

Research on the way health services are delivered and organised is part of the broader field of health services (or systems) research which has become well established in the UK, North America and parts of Europe in the last twenty years. Health services research aims to 'produce reliable and valid research data on which to base appropriate, effective, cost-effective, efficient and acceptable health services' (Bowling 1997). It is not a scientific discipline in itself but an area of applied research that draws on a range of disciplines and perspectives, including anthropology, economics, epidemiology, history, medicine, nursing, political science, sociology and statistics. It concentrates on the study of health services or systems rather than on the state of health and disease of individuals and of populations. Unlike clinical research, which has traditionally focused on individual patients in relation to their treatment and care, health services research adopts a population perspective. Questions considered by health services research include: How much health care should we have? How should services be funded? Who should receive health services? and How well are services being delivered? (Black 1997).

The interests of different stakeholders in health services have led to the growth, development and increased expectations of health services research. Funders of health care sought help to address the problem of cost containment; health care professionals, particularly doctors who have come under pressure to defend themselves against those who argued that many clinical interventions were unproven, ineffective, or even harmful (Cochrane 1972; McKeown 1979; Illich 1976), have sought scientific evidence from health services research to defend their practices; and users of health services have looked to this research to support their growing demands for more information about the care they receive.

These pressures have led to two tendencies. First, the focus of health services research has tended to be on health technology assessment (HTA). Second, the emphasis on the randomised trial, although necessary, has 'retarded the development of a broader view of evaluation' (St Leger and Walsworth-Bell 1999). This focus has, until recently, underplayed the importance of research on how health services are managed, organised and delivered. This is not to say that research on these issues has not been carried out in the last twenty years. On the contrary, many good examples of SDO research exist. Research has been conducted on different funding systems, such as different methods of paying for health care in the USA (Newhouse and the Insurance Experiment Group 1993) and general practitioner fundholding in the UK (Mays et al. 1997); the basis for resource allocation within a health care system (Carr-Hill et al. 1994); the nature of organisational structures within health systems, such as internal markets (Allen 1995); the impact of organisational change on health care providers (Shortell et al. 2000); evaluations of different models of care such as community mental health teams (Tyrer et al. 1998) and hospital-at-home services (Fulop et al. 1997); the appropriateness of the use of acute hospital beds (Victor et al. 1993); analyses of interactions between health care professionals and patients (Stimson and Webb 1975; Strong 1979); and the impact of different approaches to management, such as the impact of the introduction of general management (Strong and Robinson 1990).

There is not, of course, a clearly defined boundary between HTA and questions relating to health service delivery and organisation. Indeed, some would argue that it is a false distinction to make, as technical and organisational or social considerations are so interwoven that they should not be studied in isolation (Gibbons *et al.* 1994). SDO and HTA research complement one another. For example, HTA can provide evidence on the cost-effectiveness of one particular intervention (such as a drug or surgical technique) compared with another, while SDO research would then be required to determine, for example, where the best setting (e.g. primary or secondary care) for the delivery of that intervention would be. Other areas of SDO research include comparisons of different models of care, organisational issues at different levels (such as within teams, departments or entire organisations), and the management of change in health care organisations.

In England, while research on the delivery and organisation of services has been broadly supported in the past, it received a major boost with the establishment of a national government-funded programme in 1999 (http://www.sdo.lshtm.ac.uk). Initiatives in other countries, such as the Canadian Health Services Research Foundation (Lomas 2000) and the Australian Centre for Effective Healthcare (http://www.aceh.usyd.edu.au), have also increased the focus in this area internationally. In the USA, the Agency for Healthcare Research and Quality (http://www.ahcpr.gov) is one of a number of organisations which funds research in this area.

Some fundamentals

Given the wide range of disciplines that contribute to the field of SDO research, it is inevitable that certain methodological tensions will arise. It is important that these are recognised and understood if multidisciplinary working is to be achieved and the potential contribution of research is to be realised. This section will discuss some of these tensions and, as a preliminary matter, it is important to give working definitions of some key terms used throughout this book. These terms, such as epistemology, discipline, paradigm, approach, method and methodology, are first defined briefly below before we discuss their implications for SDO research in the remainder of this section. It should be noted that the definitions provided might seem to underestimate their complexity and contestability, but have been simplified for the purposes of this book.

Epistemology refers to a branch of philosophy concerned with the theory of knowledge. The central questions it addresses are the nature and derivation of knowledge, its scope, and the reliability of its claims. The related term *ontology* concerns what can be known, that is, the kinds of things that exist. It is important to understand the debates arising from these questions, as they have been highly influential in the development of many of the disciplines discussed in this book.

The term *paradigm* can be used to describe the 'world view' adopted by the researcher, that is, the general theoretical assumptions that members of a particular scientific or research community adopt. These may be either explicit or implicit in the researcher's work. An example of a paradigm is positivism – research based on the assumption that there is a single reality, i.e. one set of 'facts' about the world which may be observed. Thus different paradigms are based on different epistemologies.

A *discipline* is used to refer to a group of academics with an identifiable perspective or focus, such as economics or sociology. The extent to which a researcher's training leads him or her to formulate and pursue research questions in a way that differs from that expected of researchers with a different disciplinary background can usefully be considered under three headings: the questions asked, the concepts used, and the research techniques employed. Members of a discipline may all adhere to the same paradigm or to different ones. There are frequently debates within disciplines, such as sociology and psychology, because different researchers within those disciplines use what are seen as competing paradigms (see Chapters 2, 3 and 5).

In this book we use the term *approach* to describe a way of going about the research process. Action research (Chapter 11) and operational research (Chapter 10) might more accurately be described as *approaches* to research rather than as separate disciplines. Although action research draws heavily on sociology it does not do so exclusively, and operational research, which has its roots in engineering science, uses a wide variety of methods. The distinct feature for both action research and operational research is that the researcher works with those being researched, both to design research questions and to optimise and implement solutions. The disadvantage of this closer local focus is that generalisability may be compromised. The advantage is that the likelihood of appropriate implementation may be enhanced. Some would say these approaches sit on the border between research and change management, issues discussed further in Chapters 10 and 11.

The term *theory* is used in a number of ways in research and, once again, different disciplines and paradigms have contrasting perspectives on it. A theory is an explanation, explaining the phenomenon of interest (for example, 'the organisation' or 'leadership'). Theory may provide the focus for the study, an idea for investigation. It can also assist the researcher to formulate and reformulate the problem addressed by the research. A particular theory can be tested by empirical research and its limitations analysed. However, while the positivist tradition sees a clear distinction between the role of theory and data (that empirical research is used merely to test 'hypotheses', i.e. theories), other traditions posit a more complex relationship between theory and empirical research. In the latter, research shapes, initiates, reformulates and clarifies theory. An example of this approach is the notion of 'grounded theory' proposed by Glaser and Strauss (1967) whereby theory is generated and developed from the data.

Methods refer to particular techniques for undertaking research, for example the in-depth interview or the randomised controlled trial. *Methodology* refers to the general approach to undertaking research generated from within a particular paradigm in accordance with its general framework or body of theory. The term methodology may also refer to the study or science of research methods.

Methods, theories and hypotheses can be shared between disciplines or approaches. However, different theoretical approaches may provide contrasting views of the same data collection methods. For example, researchers in the positivist tradition treat interview data very differently from those from an interactionist or an interpretivist tradition (Silverman 1985).

Competing paradigms?

There are two main dimensions along which it is possible to characterise the disciplines described in this book. Broadly these are:

1   positivism/objectivity versus interactionism/interpretivism/subjectivity
2   deductive versus inductive approaches to research.

Different disciplines, and different traditions within disciplines, stem from different paradigms and theories of knowledge. Clearly these differences are important.

One of the most important dimensions is the difference between objectivity or positivism and subjectivity or interactionism. Positivism can be characterised by the assertion that 'the facts are definitely out there', they merely require gathering by the industrious researcher – that is, there is one version of reality. In contrast, an interactionist or an interpretivist works within a paradigm where an interpretation is sought for what is observed, and 'truths' or 'facts' are not 'out there' but dependent on different actors' viewpoints. Nevertheless, it is thought by some adherents of this latter view that observations can be made from which a consensus may be reached (Ovretveit 1998; Hatch 1997).

It is important to note that both 'sides' of this dimension contain a very wide range of views. There can be as many debates between those on the 'subjective side' as between, say, interactionists and positivists. Another set of ideas – postmodernist ideas – illustrates this. These ideas have been very influential in a number of disciplines in relation to questions of objectivity (see Chapters 2, 3 and 9). The huge variety of ideas labelled postmodern, and their core value of diversity, means that summarisation is not feasible or appropriate. However, there are some critical aspects which require description. Postmodernists believe that knowledge is fundamentally fragmented, that is, 'knowledge is produced in so many bits and pieces ... there can be no reasonable expectation that it will add up to an integrated and singular view'

(Hatch 1997). This leads to criticisms of efforts at universal understanding as 'grand narrative' (Lyotard 1979). Most importantly, postmodernists challenge modern notions of truth and the search for one best way to understand phenomena. Postmodernism denies the priority of observation which underpins most of modern science, and thereby opens the scientific view of knowledge for debate. Modernism is interpreted by postmodernists as a series of truth 'claims' (Hatch 1997).

Each paradigm, as we have characterised them here, presents a potential problem for SDO research. In the case of interactionism or interpretivism, for example, are the results so subjective that generalisable truths cannot be drawn about the way a service is organised independently of the particular organisation researched or the particular researcher undertaking that research? And the converse problem pertains with an entirely positivist view in which the researcher is unaware of the inextricable effect the research may be having on the very 'truths' he or she is hoping to uncover, and unaware that another researcher might derive a very different account from the same research.

It is easy to characterise these paradigms as diametrically opposed and constituting unbridgeable barriers to those who would adopt one or another – what has been termed 'paradigm wars' (Pawson and Tilley 1997). To some extent, 'positivism' has been seen as made of straw, as researchers based in a broadly positivist tradition also often recognise that observation is theory-impregnated (Popper 1972) and that knowledge is socially organised (Kuhn 1970). Similarly, researchers from other traditions have come to acknowledge the importance of being explicit about the methods used (Chapters 2 and 12). Others argue that these 'paradigm wars' have been unproductive in answering important social questions (Oakley 2000).

One perspective on scientific explanation which claims to avoid the extremes of the traditional paradigms of positivism and relativism is that of 'realism' (Pawson and Tilley 1997; Silverman 1985). This focuses on the mechanics of explanation, and how these explanatory strategies can lead to the development of a body of scientific knowledge. It has been used by some social scientists to explain social phenomena. Based within this perspective, Pawson and Tilley propose what they describe as 'an attempt at paradigm liberation' in arguing for an approach to the evaluation of social programmes called 'realistic evaluation' (Pawson and Tilley 1997).

However, others are critical of this realist approach (see Chapter 3). Hammersley (1992), for example, proposes an alternative – 'subtle realism' – to transcend the dichotomy between positivism and subjectivity/relativism. The subtle realist believes that the world exists independently of the researcher, and that it is possible to undertake research on organisations. However, he or she acknowledges that both the researcher and the organisation will inevitably be affected by the process. The research is then designed not so much to uncover 'facts' or 'truths' as to represent them accurately.

There is a recognition that other representations from a different perspective might also be possible. One would expect these representations to be complementary because all would relate to the independent, underlying reality of the situation.

A second key dimension is the difference between deductive and inductive approaches. The deductive approach is theory-driven and research is undertaken with an *a priori* theoretical view. A hypothesis is generated and, classically, the aim of the research is to falsify the hypothesis (Popper 1972). The inductive approach is data-driven – facts derived from the research are used to generate theory.

These approaches to the acquisition of knowledge lead different disciplines to hold different views about how knowledge is built up. For some disciplines there is a belief in the progressive acquisition of 'facts' or 'truths', while for others there is a more inductive approach which is not linear and where knowledge is built up through observation (Chalmers 1998; Ovretveit 1998; Guba and Lincoln 1989).

The stances taken on these two dimensions inform the way the world is viewed by each discipline. They probably account for the deepest divisions both between and within disciplines, and between researchers. Although many researchers have an awareness of the range of standpoints, their approaches to these two dimensions are likely to affect a broad range of issues relevant to their research. These include the types of research undertaken; the role of the researcher; the focus on process or outcomes; the role of context and the extent of generalisability; approaches to the issues of reliability and validity; and the types of methods used. These issues are discussed further below.

The types of research undertaken

The types of research undertaken, as we have argued, are informed by the approach researchers take to the two key dimensions discussed above. Broadly speaking, researchers closest to the positivist, deductive view tend to privilege experimentation above other types of research; while those taking an interactionist, inductive approach are more concerned with observing and describing the 'meanings' of the social world.

The gold standard for organisational psychology and for epidemiology, for example, is the controlled experiment – an experiment controlled by the researcher examining the effects of a change in service delivery imposed from outside (see Chapters 4 and 5). An experiment artificially interferes with the natural working of an organisation to test a hypothesis or a theory. Other researchers from a positivist perspective aim to build models which can then be tested. This is particularly true for operational research and organisational psychology, but can also apply in other disciplines, such as economics.

Researchers from an interactionist or interpretivist approach (such as some within the disciplines of organisational studies, sociology and policy analysis, for example) tend to use everyday or 'natural' contexts as their sources of data (see Chapters 2, 3 and 6).

Role of the researcher

A further distinction between researchers is how they view their role in the research, and this is related to another important distinction, that between formative and summative intentions. In formative research, the role of the researcher is to feed back results to those being studied as the research progresses in order to inform further change.

Action research, for example, takes a formative approach. Those under-taking action research suggest that the inevitable effect a researcher will have on an organisation or individuals while undertaking research should be harnessed for positive benefits within the organisation. In action research, implementation and research occur iteratively, and the researcher is part of the change process. This illustrates the underlying philosophy of action research (Chapter 11), as distinct from other approaches that emphasise the distinction between the role of the researcher and the phenomenon they are studying, while recognising that the research process and the phenomenon will interact with each other. Researchers from most of the other disciplines described in this book carry out research which is more summative in its intentions, aiming to produce a research result but not to undertake imple-mentation of the findings.

Processes, inputs, outputs and outcomes

A key challenge for research in health service delivery and organisation is that the phenomena under study (for example, a change to the way a service is delivered or organised) are complex and difficult to define.

A common criticism of the experimental approach is that by focusing on inputs and outputs it fails to take account both of the underlying processes and the social context within which a change is introduced. These are an inherent part of the change, and vital to understanding why it does or does not work. Some researchers therefore eschew completely the experimental method with its focus on inputs and outputs (characterised as the 'black box' approach) to focus instead on context and processes. For example, a researcher might adopt the case study method deliberately in order to study the contextual conditions of a particular phenomenon because the bound-aries between the phenomenon and its context are not clear (Yin 1994) (see Chapter 2).

Other researchers, interested in experimentation, use quasi- experiments or natural experiments. These occur when two similar organisations differ apparently only in whether or not they have adopted the change in service delivery that is the subject of the research, or where it is possible to gather data from the organisation before and after the adoption of the change. While some researchers view the lack of 'control' of the experiment as inevitably bound to confound any findings, others believe that 'natural experiments' provide a good test-bed for changes in service delivery that cannot be subjected to controlled experimentation. Still others propose a revision to the experimental approach in order to take context and processes into account (Pawson and Tilley 1997) (see Chapter 6).

Role of context: generalisability, validity and reliability

As we have argued, context is an important factor in the study of health service delivery and organisation. As we have seen, to some researchers, context is seen as a confounder, a nuisance to be factored out wherever possible. To others, context is an integral part of the texture of an organisation and, therefore, of research into that organisation and organisations in general. In the former case, context may disrupt the relationship between an intervention and its intended outcome; in the latter case, context may itself be the subject of the research, eventually allowing for a richer understanding of the generalisability of the findings.

Almost all research strives for generalisability (also referred to as external validity). Research which is never intended to be generalisable should be more accurately called audit (or monitoring or performance assessment). In contrast, research is aimed at developing or consolidating insights or understandings which can be applied across settings.

One of the challenges in SDO research is that interventions tend to be diffuse, complex and difficult to define. Disciplines differ in the approach they take to this problem. For epidemiologists, it is important in the case of a controlled trial to have a sufficiently narrow definition of the intervention. However, this runs the risk of evaluating an intervention which, although clearly and narrowly defined, fails to take account of how this intervention would operate in a day-to-day setting. For epidemiologists, a diffuse definition of the intervention may enhance the pragmatic value of the study but reduce the likelihood of explanatory power of the study. For other disciplines and approaches, such as organisational studies or policy analysis, the emphasis would be on evaluating an intervention within the context into which it has been introduced, and its 'diffuseness' would be part of the study.

Validity and reliability are closely related to the issue of generalisability. Validity (or more strictly, internal validity) is the extent to which an observation is measuring what it is intended to measure. For example, the validity of a cost estimate could be called into question if the only costs considered were those due to the use of formal services while informal care (care by friends and relations) was excluded. Reliability is the extent to which observations are repeatable in the same circumstances. However, as with the other concepts we have discussed, reliability and validity are viewed differently by different disciplines and paradigms (see Chapters 3 and 6).

An example of this is illustrated by the concept of 'triangulation'. Triangulation broadly refers to the use of multiple methods in research. There are four types of triangulation: data triangulation (different sources of data); theory triangulation (applying different perspectives to the same data source); investigator triangulation (among different researchers); and methodological triangulation (Patton 1987). However, the majority of texts referring to triangulation generally discuss the first two types. A positivist view of the triangulation of data sources or methods is that it would increase the validity of the data because, by enabling the comparison of a number of accounts, it would be able to reduce bias. For an interactionist, however, without bias (that is, a range of different accounts) there would be no phenomenon. The researcher's role, therefore, from this perspective is not 'to adjudicate between participants' competing versions' (Dingwall 1981) but to understand 'the situated work that they do' (Silverman 1985) (see Chapter 3).

Methods: qualitative and quantitative

Methods are the particular techniques used to undertake research. However, they should not be viewed separately from the fundamental debates concerning epistemology we have outlined above. There has been some debate over whether particular methods are allied to, and grounded in particular and opposing paradigms (Guba and Lincoln 1994; Oakley 2000) (see Chapter 3).

But while the adoption of either mainly qualitative or quantitative methods might be seen as one of the most important and key divisions between researchers, it is not such a deep division between disciplines. Economics, for example, is usually regarded as a quantitative discipline, but qualitative methods are often used in organisational economics (Chapter 8). Most of the disciplines represented in this book draw on both qualitative and quantitative methods. An organisational studies case study, for example, might include quantitative methods such as surveys. An example of the use of different methods from different disciplines (multidisciplinary research) is where qualitative research is used alongside a randomised trial to help understand quantitative findings.

Macro, meso and micro levels in health service delivery and organisation research

Different disciplines focus their study on the same research topic at different organisational levels. The choice of level is partly informed by theory and partly by pragmatism. If we characterise research at the level of the health system as 'macro', the 'meso' is taken here to mean at the level of institutions, and 'micro' the level of the individual practitioners or patients. Because of their theoretical base, some disciplines lend themselves to a particular level. For example, policy analysis and history tend to focus at the macro and meso levels, whereas epidemiology and organisational psychology are more suited to investigating the meso and micro levels.

Issues involved in undertaking multidisciplinary research

As we have described, there are important differences both between and within disciplines which need to be understood if multidisciplinary research is possible. Multidisciplinary work is easiest where researchers from the different disciplines share paradigms. Thus it is possible to imagine epidemiologists and economists sharing a broadly 'positivist' perspective working together to evaluate a change in the way a health service is delivered (Chapters 4 and 7). Similarly, it is possible to imagine researchers from organisational studies and policy analysis with an interpretivist perspective working together to study the same change in delivery of a health service (Chapters 2 and 6).

The key question is whether it is possible, or indeed desirable, for researchers from different paradigms to work together to address the same research problem. As we have tried to emphasise, these perspectives are not necessarily at opposite poles – they each form a range of views, along a continuum. Therefore it is possible to envisage researchers from the less extreme end of their particular continuum of the different perspectives working together. For example, it is possible to imagine a 'subtle realist' using qualitative methods to study a change in service delivery that has uniquely occurred in one organisation, while an epidemiologist uses this 'natural experiment' to compare this organisation with another one. It is also important to recognise that it will be not be possible to reconcile the more extreme positions within each perspective. It is difficult to imagine an epidemiologist working alongside a researcher from a postmodernist perspective within organisational studies.

In the final section of this chapter, we take an example of a change in service delivery (the introduction of telemedicine) and show how the different disciplines and approaches described in this book could be used to address the various research questions that arise from this change. It is up to the researchers from these disciplines and approaches to see how far they can work together to carry out research in this important area of health service delivery and organisation.

Outline of the book

In this section we describe the content and format of this book. Chapters 2–11 follow a common format, shown in Box 1.1.

Box 1.1 Format of chapters 2–11

Definition and theoretical basis of the discipline

This provides a definition of, and discusses the theoretical background to the discipline.

Uses

This discusses the *types* of research questions which can be addressed by this discipline and which types of research questions it would not be appropriate for.

How to undertake the discipline

Includes data sources, data collection methods and data analysis, and gives examples of where this discipline has contributed or could contribute to research in health service delivery and organisation.

Limitations

Discusses the limitations of the discipline's contribution.

Further reading

We start by considering sociological approaches. These can be used at both the meso (organisational) level and at the micro level. Chapter 2 on organisational studies explains that it is a social science discipline which has grown out of its original base in sociology. Its focus is the meso level – formally constituted organisations and their importance as a site for social action. In organisational studies (unlike neo-classical economics), behaviour of individuals and organisations is viewed as 'socially embedded' through such factors as norms, culture, and power relations. Key themes within organisational studies which can be applied to health care include: organisational change and continuity; organisational culture; and changes to the division of organisational labour. In contrast, qualitative sociology at the micro level, discussed in Chapter 3, explores interactions between individuals within health care settings. The theoretical and epistemological basis of this methodology is highly contested, and these debates are outlined. These methods can be used to undertake studies in inaccessible settings; to provide rigorous descriptions; to generate hypotheses; to explain unexpected findings and negative cases; and to infer participants' meanings.

We then consider one of the quantitative disciplines used in SDO research: epidemiology. Chapter 4 shows how epidemiological techniques can be applied to organisational problems in health services, particularly the evaluation of interventions. In contrast to most of the disciplines discussed in this book, these methods (in common with economic evaluation) concentrate on the comparison of the outcomes of different modes of service delivery or organisational structures, as opposed to studying the processes themselves. The pre-eminence of the randomised controlled trial (RCT) is explained, and the use of cluster randomisation is also described. The use of non-randomised study designs, including time series analyses and cohort studies, is also discussed.

Next we look at the contribution of organisational psychology. Chapter 5 discusses the way in which this discipline is essentially quantitative and concerned with the behaviour, thoughts and emotions of individuals and groups within organisations. The focus on the individual is similar to that of micro-sociology, although the use of quantitative data is not. The chapter describes the advantages and limitations of such a positivist, quantitative approach. Key themes within organisational psychology which can be applied to health care include teamwork, stress and burnout, motivation, career progression and leadership.

Chapter 6, on policy analysis, explains how it is rooted in the discipline of political science. The major concern is with questions of the cleavages of interest between 'actors', inequalities in power between them and the ways in which differences of interest are mediated (i.e. the political process). This chapter describes how policy analysis uses these concepts to focus on the processes by which policies are made, the context in which this occurs, and how policy analysis can be applied to the organisation and delivery of services. Unlike micro-sociological methods, this approach works at a relatively high level of aggregation and would not be suitable for investigating detailed questions about how individuals are interacting. It overlaps with organisational studies in its interest in how policies are implemented at local level.

Economic analysis can be used in two ways to research the delivery and organisation of health services. The first is in answering normative questions about how resources should be allocated between different interventions or modes of delivery, and the second is in analysing and describing the effect of different organisational forms.

Chapter 7 on economic evaluation explains how this formal quantitative economic technique is concerned with questions about the efficient allocation of resources. It can be used to compare alternative courses of action in terms of their costs and consequences. In order to make such comparisons, economic evaluation employs a single measure of benefit, which is usually a state of health. For questions concerning the organisation and delivery of services, there may be more than one relevant benefit, as not all organisational changes are designed simply to improve health. Other disciplines, such as policy analysis, may have to be employed in conjunction with economic evaluation.

Chapter 8 on organisational economics complements that on economic evaluation, explaining how interest in this discipline focuses on the effects on costs of different ways of organising the production of services (or products) and of organising their exchange between organisations. This type of economic analysis is relevant to questions such as the appropriateness of boundaries between organisations, and the incentives that influence the behaviour of individuals when responding to scarcity. As organisational economics is based on theory concerning opportunity cost, it is not primarily concerned with issues such as the context in which organisations operate.

The value of historical research to the provision of contemporary health care is not usually recognised. In Chapter 9, the eclectic nature of history and the way it has been perceived as atheoretical is discussed. Historical research is particularly suited to analysing change (e.g. how current organisational structures and modes of delivery of care resemble or differ from previous ones). However, it cannot be used to answer evaluative questions about 'what works?'.

Operational research is a process of offering aid to organisational decision-making through the construction of models representing the interaction of relevant factors, which can be used to clarify the implications of choice (Chapter 10). It has principally been concerned with quantitative modelling of practical problems in health services – for example in the application of queuing theory to waiting lists and appointment timings. However, newer qualitative techniques are becoming more prevalent and are also described in this chapter. Operational research is not primarily designed to answer evaluative questions about what works, but to clarify the consequences of alternative actions.

Action research (Chapter 11) may be described as an approach rather than a discipline. It derives insights from naturally occurring data collected by the researcher who is involved in the processes of interest. Its distinctive feature is that it requires the researcher to intervene in the setting to be studied. By working with and for, rather than on people, it aims to bridge the gap between research and practice. Action research is a formative process whereby results are continuously fed back in order to achieve further change. In contrast to disciplines such as economics and sociology, action researchers are less concerned with the need to generate a knowledge base through generalisation, and more interested in the facilitation of change in specific settings. Any organisational process in health care can be subjected to this approach, and examples include lay participation in care on hospital wards, and partnerships between organisations.

Finally, in Chapter 12, methods of synthesising SDO research evidence are discussed. In contrast to much previous work on the synthesis of experimentally derived, quantitative data (about which there is some consensus) there are difficulties concerning epistemological and methodological standpoints, which render synthesis of non-experimental quantitative and qualitative studies problematic. In addition, there are related issues about the quality of evidence. The chapter recommends that it is generally better to use quality criteria to determine the weight to be given to particular studies in drawing conclusions, rather than strict inclusion or exclusion criteria. Fine judgements will be required at every stage of a synthesis of evidence of this type, and the chapter suggests that evidence should be synthesised in a 'scholarly' rather than a technical way.

A worked case example

So far we have outlined the various disciplines and theoretical approaches that may be used to study the delivery and organisation of health services. In this section, we show how these different disciplines and approaches might be applied, in various combinations, to specific research questions.

As a way of thinking about this, imagine a group of health care practitioners and managers who are concerned to improve services for orthopaedic patients. Practitioners and managers require research evidence on a number of different aspects of the way such services are delivered and organised, to ensure the best possible service is provided within the resources available. The questions they need to ask are:

- What is the best way of delivering orthopaedic care?
- Having identified the best way, how can change in existing services be implemented?
- How can care be improved further by means of organisational change?

For each of these questions, we illustrate how the various disciplines and methods discussed in this book could be used to address specific research questions. We have taken as a given that, prior to any empirical research being undertaken, any necessary synthesis of existing research has been carried out, along the lines outlined in Chapter 12.

At the interface between primary and secondary care, managers first want to improve communication between practitioners so as to enhance patient care. In particular, they might want to know whether they should introduce a system of tele-orthopaedics within primary care. This system would provide a consultation and diagnostic service for GPs and their patients in the GP's surgery from orthopaedic specialists in a hospital setting. The research would need to compare the tele-orthopaedics system with the traditional model of service organisation, i.e. the patient attending a hospital outpatient clinic.

Assuming that the research shows that tele-orthopaedics as a technology is potentially a superior model of delivery to the standard one, the orthopaedic managers would then want to know how best to introduce this new system, i.e. how to implement change in health service delivery and organisation.

Finally, the managers want to take a 'whole system' approach to improving care for orthopaedic patients. They want to see how they can improve the level of integration and commitment that patients receive from the different providers in primary care, secondary care (outpatients and inpatients) and social care.

Stage one: What is the best way of delivering orthopaedic care?

Introducing a tele-orthopaedics service would allow general practitioners to obtain an orthopaedic opinion in their own surgery rather than refer patients to the hospital outpatient department. While the new service would mean that patients, many of whom have impaired mobility and are elderly, would not have to travel to obtain an orthopaedic opinion, there are several uncertainties regarding the potential impact of this new way of organising and delivering a service. Will it be as effective in terms of accuracy of diagnosis? Will it be as efficient for the health service, given the initial capital investment and the GP's time involved in tele-consultations? What impact might telemedicine have on the relationship between the GP and the specialist? What impact might it have on the patient's relationship with both the GP and the specialist? At least four disciplines could help answer these questions: epidemiology, economics, history and sociology.

Will telemedicine be as clinically effective in terms of accuracy of diagnosis? (epidemiological research)

It may be possible to carry out a randomised trial in which patients needing an orthopaedic opinion are randomly allocated either to be referred to the hospital outpatient department or to be seen in the GP's surgery via the telemedicine link to the hospital. It would be necessary to recruit a sufficient number of GPs prepared to randomise their patients. Given that telemedicine is a new service, it could be decided that it was only available within the trial. Thus GPs or patients not wishing to be randomised would be referred to outpatients in the traditional way. Effectiveness would be assessed as the proportion of patients who were correctly diagnosed, as judged independently by another orthopaedic surgeon who was unaware which form of consultation had occurred. This is the kind of trial suited to cluster randomisation, because if a GP has access to the telemedicine service, this might inadvertently affect the way that he or she manages the 'control' patients. This is known as 'contamination'. Cluster randomisation where, for example, GP practices rather than individual patients are randomised, reduces this risk of contamination though it increases the size of the sample needed for the study.

Will telemedicine be as efficient for the health service? (economic evaluation)

As well as assessing the relative effectiveness of telemedicine, an economic evaluation could also be conducted. The costs of both types of consultation would need to be determined. The principal additional costs for telemedicine would be a contribution to the capital cost of the equipment, the cost of transmission of images and the GP's time. The orthopaedic surgeon's time and the cost of investigations might be the same as for consultation at the outpatient department, though this cannot be assumed. Both would need to be measured in both arms of the trial. The difference in costs borne by the patients and their families when using telemedicine or conventional care would need to be measured. All these costs could be collected during the randomised trial.

What impact might telemedicine have on the relationship between the GP and the specialist? (historical research)

Some people have voiced concern that telemedicine might adversely affect the long-standing relationship between general practitioners and specialists. Others have suggested the converse, that both parties would benefit from the joint consultations that are a feature of telemedicine. The nature of the existing relationship is the product of many years, going back to the apothecaries and barber-surgeons of medieval times. Historical research could throw light on the nature of the relationship and how it has developed, thus increasing our understanding of the impact of bringing the specialist into the GP's consulting room by means of a television link, in the presence of the patient.

What impact might telemedicine have on the patient's relationship
with the GP and the specialist? (micro-sociology)

The effectiveness (and, as a result, cost-effectiveness) of consultations
depends partly on the nature of the relationship between the doctor and the
patient. The relationship can facilitate or impede communication and understanding, and can determine the extent to which the patient participates in
decisions concerning treatment and management of their condition. It seems
likely that teleconsultations will affect the relationship a patient has with
their GP. This might be beneficial or adverse. Qualitative research using
observational methods (audio or video recording of consultations), together
with in-depth interviews of the participants, could help our understanding
of the impact of teleconsultations on the humanity of care from the
patient's perspective, and on the doctor's perception of his or her relationship with the patient.

Stage two: How can change to existing services be implemented?

If research showed that tele-orthopaedics was a better method than the
traditional model, the next step would be to use research to understand how
the delivery of services could be changed to include telemedicine. The
research question therefore concerns the investigation and evaluation of
methods to implement changes in how services are delivered.

What effect would the method of funding orthopaedic services have
on implementing telemedicine? (organisational economics)

An analysis of the financial incentives relevant to the delivery of
orthopaedic services within a hospital could be carried out. This could identify, for example, whether the hospital would lose income if, instead of
patients attending the outpatient department, they consulted with the
orthopaedic surgeon by means of telemedicine. If that were the case, there
would be an incentive for hospital managers to block the introduction of
telemedicine, unless the hospital were able concomitantly to reduce its costs
to take account of any reduction in income.

What impact will telemedicine have on the functioning of the
orthopaedic service? (operational research)

Modelling the effects on the organisation of care in the hospital as a whole,
if the desired change to telemedicine consultations were to be implemented,
could take account of changes in the use of space, or effects on waiting
times for outpatient appointments and surgery. This could pinpoint problems which might arise in the health system as telemedicine was introduced.

What impact does telemedicine have on the behaviour, attitudes
and emotions of clinical staff? (organisational psychology)

Theoretical models concerning how people learn and how they can be
induced to change their behaviour could be used to understand the relevant
aspects of the orthopaedic surgeons' personalities, motivation and cognitive
processes, in order to facilitate change. These models could be used to design
a survey of the surgeons to find out what motivational factors are most relevant in changing behaviour in these circumstances.

What happens in practice when implementation is attempted?
(action research)

By working with people involved in implementing change, action researchers
would aim to bridge the gap between theory and practice by continuously
feeding back results to the staff in the hospital in order to achieve further
change. Researchers could be part of a steering group charged with introducing telemedicine into the hospital. They could contribute by studying
and reporting on how GPs and hospital clinicians were reacting to the
proposed change.

Stage three: How can care be improved further by changes at the organisational level?

The hospital managers and practitioners now want to improve the overall
quality of care patients receive from the different component organisations –
primary care, secondary care (outpatients and inpatients) and social care –
and how a more integrated service can be provided.

Whichever discipline or combination of disciplines is used, one key
conceptual task would be to unpack the term 'integration' and arrive at definitions which could be used in the study. This might be a focus of the early
part of any study.

What incentives exist to encourage integration and what is the cost
of greater integration? (organisational economics)

The first question concerns the incentives that may exist, or not, for individuals and/or organisations to provide integrated services, both within and
across organisations. These incentives may be either financial or non-financial;
for example, a performance indicator for the hospital could be used to
encourage it to provide integrated services. A qualitative study could be
designed to analyse these incentives. The second question concerns the costs
of integration, particularly in terms of the opportunity costs of providing
integrated orthopaedic services, in other areas of health and social care. This

would involve applying theories of organisational economics to compare costs of different organisational forms.

What factors facilitate or hinder integration of services? (organisational studies)

An important aspect of organisational studies is that it emphasises the importance of *context* in understanding organisational behaviour. Although this can make generalisation difficult, organisational studies can help us understand what it is about a particular context that, for example, facilitates the integration of services. Looking at a range of hospitals, case studies could identify organisational factors that facilitate or hinder integration of services. These factors might include organisational form and the organisational division of labour. For example, does the integration of organisations providing orthopaedic services result in improved service integration? Have some organisations been more successful at breaking down professional barriers and creating multidisciplinary teams to improve service integration?

Which policies might facilitate greater integration? (policy analysis)

This approach could be used to provide an analysis of key actors' values and perceptions of service integration and how better integration might be achieved. Key actors would include practitioners, managers, policy makers, planners and service users. The analysis could be used to create an 'ideal type' model of how service integration might be achieved in an ideal world, or used to compare different actors' 'framing' of the issue and compare their perceptions with any available evidence. This would aid understanding of the issues in integrating services and what issues might arise in any proposed policy intervention.

Policy analysis could also be used to evaluate particular policy interventions designed to improve integration of services. The study design might consist of comparative case studies or 'natural experiments'. Where a policy was introduced universally, the comparative case study approach could be used to compare the different contexts within which the intervention had been introduced (e.g. doctor-led or nurse-led; urban or rural setting). In the situation where a policy was not introduced universally, the comparative case study approach could compare areas where the policy had been introduced with those where it had not. In either case, such a study would seek to generalise the research findings not through aggregation, but rather through the development of theory.

This case study demonstrates the need to use a broad range of disciplines and approaches to answer the types of questions posed by SDO research. This book aims to describe and explain the contributions of a series of disciplines and approaches which will be useful to researchers and research funders in this field.

References

Allen, P. (1995) 'Contracts in the NHS internal market', *Modern Law Review*, 58: 321–42.

Black, N. (1997) 'Health services research: saviour or chimera?', *Lancet*, 349: 1834–6.

Bowling, A. (1997) *Research Methods in Health: Investigating Health and Health Services*, Buckingham: Open University Press.

Carr-Hill, R. A., Sheldon, T. A., Smith, P., Martin, S., Peacock, S. and Hardman, G. (1994) 'Allocating resources to health authorities: development of method for small area analysis of use of inpatient services', *British Medical Journal*, 309: 1046–9.

Chalmers, A. F. (1998) *What is this thing called science?*, 3rd edn, Buckingham: Open University Press.

Dingwall, R. (1981) 'The ethnomethodological movement', in G. Payne, R. Dingwall, J. Payne and M. Carter (eds) *Sociology and Social Research*, London: Croom Helm.

Fulop, N., Hood, S. and Parsons, S. (1997) 'Does the National Health Service want hospital at home?', *Journal of the Royal Society of Medicine*, 90: 212–15.

Gibbons, M., Limoges, C., Nowotny, H., Schwartzman, S., Scott, P. and Trow, M. (1994) *The New Production of Knowledge*, London: Sage.

Glaser, B. G. and Strauss, A. L. (1967) *The Discovery of Grounded Theory: Strategies for Qualitative Research*, New York: Aldine.

Guba, E. G. and Lincoln, Y. S. (1989) *Fourth Generation Evaluation*, Newbury Park CA: Sage.

Guba, E. G. and Lincoln, Y. S. (1994) 'Competing paradigms in qualitative research', in N. K. Denzin and Y. S. Lincoln (eds) *Handbook of Qualitative Research*, Thousand Oaks CA: Sage.

Hammersley, M. (1992) *What's Wrong with Ethnography?*, London: Routledge.

Hatch M. (1997) *Organisation Theory: Modern Symbolic and Postmodern Perspectives*, Oxford: Oxford University Press.

Illich, I. (1976) *Medical Nemesis: Limits to Medicine*, Harmondsworth: Penguin.

Kuhn T. (1970) *The Structure of Scientific Revolutions*, Chicago: University of Chicago Press.

Lomas, J. (2000) 'Using "linkage and exchange" to move research into policy at a Canadian foundation', *Health Affairs*, 19, 3: 236–40.

Lyotard, J. F. (1979) *The Postmodern Condition: A Report on Knowledge*, Manchester: Manchester University Press.

Mays, N., Goodwin, N., Bevan, G. and Wykes, S. (on behalf of the Total Purchasing National Evaluation Team) (1997) *Total Purchasing: a Profile of National Pilot Projects*, London: Kings Fund.

McKeown, T. (1979) *The Role Of Medicine*, 2nd edn, Oxford: Oxford University Press.

Newhouse, J. P. and the Insurance Experiment Group (1993) *Free for All? Lessons from the RAND Health Insurance Experiment*, Cambridge MA: Harvard University Press.

Oakley, A. (2000) *Experiments in Knowing*, Cambridge: Polity Press.

Ovretveit, J. (1998) *Evaluating Health Interventions*, Buckingham: Open University Press.

Patton, M. Q. (1987) *How to Use Qualitative Methods in Evaluation*, Newbury Park CA: Sage.

Pawson, R. and Tilley, N. (1997) *Realistic Evaluation*, London: Sage.

Popper, K. R. (1972) *The Logic of Scientific Discovery*, London: Hutchinson.

Relman, A. S. (1988) 'Assessment and accountability: the third revolution in medical care', *New England Journal of Medicine*, 319, 18: 1220–2.

Shortell, S. M., Jones, R. H., Rademaker, A. W., Gillies, R. R., Dranove D. S., Hughes, E. F. X., Budetti, P. P., Reynolds, K. S. E. and Huang, C. (2000) 'Assessing the impact of total quality management and organisational culture on multiple outcomes of care for coronary artery bypass graft surgery patients', *Medical Care*, 38, 2: 207–17.

Silverman, D. (1985) *Qualitative Methodology and Sociology*, Aldershot: Gower.

Stimson, G. and Webb, B. (1975) *Going to see the Doctor*, London: Routledge.

St Leger, A. S. and Walsworth Bell, J. P. (1999) *Change-Promoting Research for Health Services*, Buckingham: Open University Press.

Strong, P. (1979) *The Ceremonial Order of the Clinic: Parents, Doctors and Medical Bureaucracies*, London: Routledge and Kegan Paul.

Strong, P. and Robinson, J. (1990) *The NHS: Under New Management*, Milton Keynes: Open University Press.

Tyrer, P., Evans, K., Gandhi, N., Lamont, A., Harrison-Read, P. and Johnson, T. (1998) 'Randomised controlled trial of two models of care for discharged psychiatric patients', *British Medical Journal*, 316: 106–9.

Victor, C. R., Nazareth, B., Hudson, M. and Fulop, N. (1993) 'Inappropriate use of acute hospital beds in an inner London health authority', *Health Trends*, 25: 94–7.

Yin, R. K. (1994) *Case Study Research: Design and Methods*, 2nd edn, London: Sage.

Chapter 2

Organisational studies

Ewan Ferlie

Introduction

Health care is usually organised in large and complex systems in which many decisions are implemented across organisational layers, occupational and professional groupings. An *organisation* can be defined as an institutionalised grouping of persons which has a common structure or governance arrangement. Health care purchasers, hospitals and primary care practices are all organisations: by contrast, informal or lay care is not provided through organisations.

In practice, much health care is delivered through large and complex organisations, both on the provider side (hospitals, primary care practices) and the purchaser side (government, health maintenance organisations, insurers). An important distinction can be made between the *formal organisation* (the formal structure, lines on an organisation chart, espoused strategy) and the *informal organisation* (how staff really behave, emergent strategy). The concept of the informal organisation is often used within organisational analysis to reflect differences between the espoused and the apparent pattern of behaviour. Given the continuing presence of complex health care organisations, the question arises as to how they can best be studied.

Definition and theoretical basis

Organisational studies as a discipline has grown out of organisational sociology. Compared with psychology or micro-level sociology, it typically operates at a higher level of aggregation than the individual, the small team or the study of doctor/patient interactions. An organisation may be defined as a particular setting (such as an outpatients clinic), a large producing unit (such as a hospital) or an organisational field (the population of hospitals). Organisational studies operates at a relatively high level of analysis, between the meso and the macro level. However, it is less macro than disciplines such as political science, which often concentrate on system-wide institutions rather than local settings, or macro-sociology which analyses whole social systems.

Organisational studies is interested in how people behave within organisations, seeing such behaviour as socially embedded through such forces as norms, culture, power relations and institutions. Its founder was the German sociologist Max Weber (Runciman 1978), whose theories of bureaucratisation and charismatic leadership are still used. In America, important work was done by the Chicago School sociologists of the 1950s, much of it within health care (Becker *et al.* 1961; Goffman 1961; Strauss *et al.* 1964). Early British research was undertaken by 1960s industrial sociologists, such as Joan Woodward (1965) and the Aston Group (Pugh 1997). Since 1980 the discipline has expanded in numbers and in range, propelled by the growth of business schools.

Organisational studies displays its own internal dynamics and debates, reflecting the trends observable within the social sciences as a whole. There are emerging feminist, neo-Marxist and postmodernist subgroups alongside more orthodox groupings. A recent overview (Clegg *et al.* 1996) suggests that there is not one organisation theory but many. For example, American organisational studies tend to the positivistic ('fact' oriented) and functionalist (designed to improve managerial performance); European organisational studies are more critical (anti-managerial or neo-Marxist) and theorised (for example, using postmodernist perspectives), and British organisational studies occupy an intermediary position. Organisational studies is not therefore defined by any particular theory it espouses or methods it employs.

But what kind of discipline is it? Compared with the natural sciences, organisational studies is more grounded in an explicit theoretical position. Value neutrality has been traditionally prized within natural science. However, Cooke (1999) has traced strong underlying values that lie behind the work of well known organisational authors such as Kurt Lewin and Edgar Schein. Some organisational researchers are committed to particular values rather than to neutrality, proclaiming the emancipatory role of research for lower-level participants by exploring – and exposing – organisational power.

Finally, organisational studies is often contextual in orientation, based on the premise that organisational behaviour can only be understood in context. There are, hence, limits to the generalisations that can be made across time periods or geographical boundaries. There is, nevertheless, a strong empirical tradition often using case study methods where the concern is more for ensuring internal validity (an accurate picture of events, relations or perceptions within the case study site) rather than external validity (the ability to generalise from the case to the population of organisations).

Organisational studies has a number of similarities with policy analysis (see Chapter 6 in this volume). For example, both disciplines emphasise the study of decision making; the importance of context; the development of middle range theory (that is, a level of theory which lies between very high-level abstractions on the one hand and concrete examples on the other); and the need to pay attention to values as well as 'facts'. Some key explanatory concepts (agenda setting; non-decision making; symbolic action) are common across the two disciplines. One difference is that policy analysis has strong roots within political science and thus has a particular interest in the role of the state, particularly at the higher (ministerial) levels. This policy analytic orientation is well adapted to the study of public sector organisations where government retains a shaping role. However, in some countries, much health care is provided by the private sector, where the assumption that government strongly shapes decisions does not apply. In contrast, organisational studies is better adapted to handle the analysis of firms or discrete organisations rather than governments, springing as it does from organisational sociology. Within the health care context, organisational studies is interested in characterising health care organisations as highly *professionalised* organisations (Mintzberg 1979) as well as organisations situated within the public sector. There are then some important non-state actors (including social movements or consumer lobbies) which shape the nature of health care organisations and which need to be considered.

Uses of organisational studies

Organisational studies examines behaviour within organisational settings, including such themes as decision making, implementation and innovation. It should be remembered that there is a strong scholarly tradition in these fields, as well as normative or 'guru'-based work which is more immediately visible. There has been, for example, some fifty years of scholarly work on the management of change, going back to the seminal work of Kurt Lewin (1951). The following are the high-level research themes which are well addressed from an organisational studies perspective.

Organisational change and continuity

Patterns and processes of órganisational change represent a key strand within organisational analysis (Pettigrew *et al.* 1992) and one with high policy relevance. Authors wedded to the key role of management in organisations conceive the management of change as taking place through planned and purposive interventions, with various models of change management apparent. More critical authors explore the limits to top-down and planned change, and emphasise the unintended and emergent nature of organisational change. Such research is often of a longitudinal nature, where the identification of time periods or phasing within change becomes a critical

issue (Weick and Quinn 1999). Understanding the inhibitors to change may
be as important as identifying levers for change.

Exploring the implementation and impact of corporate change
programmes (including Total Quality Management [TQM] and Business
Process Reengineering [BPR]) represents an important addition to this literature. There is a growing literature on non-incremental forms of change
such as organisational transformation, stepwise change, breakthrough
change and centrally led change. A long-term objective should be the development of generic knowledge about implementation of large-scale efforts to
effect change.

Organisational culture

There is increased interest in the impact of organisational culture(s) on decision making (Schein 1985), raising the question of how to explore and assess
organisational culture empirically. Some authors (Peters and Waterman
1982) see 'strong' cultures as the key to high organisational performance,
and suggest that such cultures can be engineered by symbolic management
(that is, attempts to manage organisational culture through the use of the
desired symbols of that culture, such as the adoption of new forms of
speech or modes of dress by management). The exploration of highly patho-
logical organisational cultures may also be of interest. Some argue that large
organisations are characterised by multiple contrasting subcultures. More
radical writers argue that organisational 'culture' is too anaemic a term and
prefer to use the concept of 'ideology', with a clearer link to the exploration
of dominant power structures.

Changes to the division of organisational labour

The re-division of organisational labour is another important theme within
organisational studies, such as the role and power base of professional
workers (Mintzberg 1979) and their changing relationship with management
(Brock et al. 1999). Such work studies whether there is evidence of underlying processes of managerialisation or deprofessionalisation. Such work
can investigate whether traditional boundaries between occupational groups
are breaking down, with the development of stronger multidisciplinary
teams. The behaviour of the strategic apex of health care organisations is of
interest within studies of corporate governance (Ferlie et al. 1996), particularly the question of whether management boards are taking on a more
empowered role.

New organisational forms

The rise of new organisational forms within health care is an important
theme. It may be that 'Fordist' organisational forms based on mass

production of a limited range of goods may be giving way to 'post-Fordist' forms based on greater specialisation and flexibility. Within the private sector we see the growth of small and medium enterprises, with waves of delayering and downsizing of large organisations. Such enterprises are linked more through networks than traditional hierarchies. More powerful IT systems provide a novel mode of coordination, through electronically based performance management systems. The Japanese provide alternative managerial models (such as 'lean production') different from the Anglo-American models we are familiar with. Writers also proclaim the emergence of new types of organisation, such as the 'learning organisation' (Senge 1990).

How to undertake organisational studies

This section reviews methods used in organisational studies, using a recent overview of the field (Clegg *et al.* 1996) to structure the discussion. A basic distinction is between quantitative and qualitative paradigms. The term 'paradigm' implies that they are incommensurable: that mixing them is like trying to mix oil and water (although other researchers argue for mixed methods). Clegg and colleagues suggest that the main shift within the discipline has been from a functionalist paradigm (based on the assumptions of 'normal' science) to an interpretive paradigm that accords particular attention to questions of meaning (see Chapter 1). Associated with this shift has been a drift from quantitative methods (such as surveys) to qualitative methods (such as case studies). This shift is partial, and diverse methods coexist within organisational studies.

The present discussion uses the categories developed by Stablein (1996) to plot research methods within organisational studies as a whole (in the UK context, Bryman [1992] provides a further helpful overview).

What are the signs and symptoms of research quality in organisational studies? This is a contested area in which there may be little agreement among scholars. Nor is it likely that research quality can be simply ordered in a hierarchical and hegemonic fashion. Nevertheless, it is helpful to consider what might be taken as indicators of research quality. They do not represent candidate 'gold standards' (which would imply unwarranted methodological hegemony) but are presented as four possible indicators. They are presented here to provoke further debate: they have no further status than the author's opinion.

- *Connection to theory*: high-quality work is not solely empirical but accesses, uses and indeed develops organisational theory.
- *Explicitness of method*: high-quality work is explicit about the methods used and why; it possesses an underlying theory of method.
- *Independence of the researcher*: research work is more likely to be of high quality when it is undertaken by an independent and external

researcher that is better placed to resist 'capture' by the many vested interests in the field.

- *Substantial empirical base*: high-quality work should provide a substantial empirical base if it is to influence policy. Concerns for generalisation and replication can be addressed in a number of ways: a preference for multiple rather than single case studies; initial case study work can be complemented by wider surveys; it suggests the creation of alliances between teams so that there are replication studies; the use of personal overviews of related sets of studies is encouraged; and 'upscaling' the empirical base.

Quantitative organisational studies

Despite Clegg and colleagues' observations, quantitative organisational research lives on, especially in the USA and in applied forms of research (such as market research directly sponsored by health care or other organisations, designed to elicit consumer views) which often use survey methods. Donaldson (1996) defends the paradigm of organisational studies as 'normal science' where positivistic methods are appropriate. Comparative survey methods may be used, in which organisations are plotted along various dimensions, using a quantitative scale or series of ordered categories. These data are coded and analysed using correlation statistics or modelling techniques (such as multiple regression). There are concerns to ensure generalisability of findings through replication.

Quantitative methods have produced classic works, such as the Aston Group studies in the 1960s of the organisational structure of firms (Pugh 1997). The Aston Group developed a large number of instruments to measure the underlying dimensions of organisations (in fact, firms) such as the degree of centralisation and formalisation, with attention to the reliability of these instruments. They used modelling techniques (such as multiple regression) to predict organisational structure from their questionnaire data and knowledge of the firms in their sample. Other authors applied this contingency theoretical approach to predict the rate of innovation in health and welfare organisations from other variables (Aiken and Hage 1971). Others have investigated the impact of managerial interventions on health care quality (Box 2.1).

Questionnaires and survey methods

The questionnaire may be the single most popular method used within organisational studies. Questionnaires can be highly structured in nature (using formal scales such as Likert scales) or be looser, relying on open-ended questions or verbatim text. They are frequently used for the collection of 'countable' data. The mailed survey is used to gather basic descriptive

Box 2.1 The impact of Total Quality Management on clinical performance

This is a well conducted example of a largely quantitative design applied to the study of American hospitals. The researchers explored whether there was any evidence of impact of TQM on general organisational culture or on outcomes of coronary artery bypass graft (CABG) surgery. This study attempted to link intermediate indicators of organisational process with final clinical outcomes. It was a prospective cohort study of 3,045 eligible CABG patients using risk-adjusted outcomes. Implementation of TQM was measured by a 58-item instrument based on Likert scales. The organisational culture section of the questionnaire used a 20-item instrument in which respondents assigned 100 total points to four possible dimensions of culture. The data were analysed by modelling techniques. The presence of TQM programmes and a supportive organisational culture were not significantly associated with differences in many quality and clinical outcome variables.

(Shortell et al. 2000)

information about populations of health care organisations, either cross-sectionally or longitudinally on a time series basis. Such techniques are good at capturing structural data (for example, membership of boards of management or the formal committee structure) but poorly adapted to handle more nuanced data (for example, where on the board does power really lie?).

Experimental comparative methods

There is greater use of experimental comparative methods within organisational research than one might think. The randomised trial with double-blind randomisation is rarely used or practicable (see Chapter 4) but non-randomised comparisons may be feasible (Campbell and Stanley 1966).

Within non-randomised comparisons, two matched sets of health care organisations may be compared (one set receives a management 'intervention'; the other does not) and the impact on outcomes is assessed (Box 2.2). This tradition is weak within UK organisational studies. Qualitative researchers contest the utility of this approach, where the intervention or technology being evaluated is highly diffuse. For example, an evaluation of TQM found a high degree of local customisation so that the 'intervention' was disparate in nature (Joss and Kogan 1995). The difficulty of matching

Box 2.2 Matching resources to needs in community care

This was a carefully designed non-randomised comparison of a new form of community care organisation (a social work team with greater flexibility and budgetary delegation) for the care of the frail elderly compared to the traditional approach. The innovative team was based in one area of England and was compared against the standard service available in a neighbouring area with a similar social and demographic profile. The sample was made up of seventy-four carefully matched pairs of elderly clients (one member of which was based in each site). The selection process included attempts to ensure similar referral and exclusion procedures, and also the use of post-selection matching.

Clinical and social outcome measures were used to plot clients' outcomes over time. In this way, the additional effectiveness of the innovative service as against the standard service was assessed. The costs of the two forms of service were assessed. A descriptive analysis of the social work activity undertaken within the new service (based on a then novel model of case management) was also undertaken, which provided an explanation of what was going on to produce such enhanced outcomes.

(Davies and Challis 1986)

and the inability to contain extraneous factors may make such designs difficult to implement in practice.

Secondary data

Such data include routinely generated employment figures, annual reports and production figures. Such data are generated for managerial purposes and may be of poor quality from a research point of view. They may be used in applied managerial evaluations, such as those carried out by inspectoral or regulatory bodies. They have a secondary use within research, used in a complementary way over and above primary data. A study in the UK of the implementation of Business Process Reengineering included data routinely generated in addition to primary data collection (Bowns and McNulty 1999). In the 1990s there was explosive growth in applied managerial evaluations, which are still increasingly being requested by policy makers, although their methodological base is often poor. The time and cost constraints often encountered may produce a research style which has been summarised as 'poverty in pragmatism' (Mark and Dopson 1999).

Qualitative organisational studies

Clegg and colleagues (1996) argue that the key trend within organisational studies has been the erosion of the functionalist paradigm, typically based on quantitative data collection. Instead, a plethora of alternative approaches has emerged using a combination of interpretive, sense-making, phenomenological, neo-Marxist or postmodernist approaches. Qualitative research has a long history within organisational studies, going back to the early work of the Chicago School of urban sociology. It assumes (Denzin and Lincoln 1994) an emphasis on processes and meanings, rather than measurement. Such researchers investigate how social experience is constructed and given meaning within particular social contexts, in an anthropological tradition. Organisational studies continues to be strongly influenced by these qualitative traditions, as do other social sciences (see Chapter 3).

Ethnography

Ethnography is a major method within organisational studies, where 'ethno researchers' are intent on discovering and communicating an organisational reality as experienced by inhabitants of that reality. In place of using ready-made constructs, the researcher's task is to discover constructs in data, often through the use of emergent or grounded theory (themes or constructs emerge from the primary data through increasingly sophisticated analysis). This method was a popular tool in the analysis of socially deviant groups (such as prisoners, delinquents and mental hospital patients) undertaken by Chicago School sociologists. The quality of such data is associated with the fidelity with which it represents these organisational worlds. There may be several such worlds, associated with different occupational groups or subcultures. Methods often used include non-participant and participant observation, which produce ethnographies (in-depth descriptions of organisational life) (Box 2.3). Observation at meetings and the analysis of documentary materials are also important methods. Where interviews do

---

Box 2.3 An ethnography of a psychiatric hospital

This single-case ethnography was based on participant observation methods where the researcher worked in a psychiatric hospital for a year as a medical administrator, and thereby gained access to what was really happening in the hospital, which differed markedly from officially produced accounts. He achieved intensive and repeated observation of patterns of patient/doctor interaction, but his main

> focus was on the role of the institution. His research can be best
> seen as a lived experience. He produced data from a grounded theo-
> retical perspective that was theorised into the concept of a total
> institution, which produced patterns of institutionalised behaviour.
>
> (Goffman 1961)

occur, they may be relatively unstructured and led by the respondent rather than the researcher. Measuring a particular dimension is less important than portraying the gestalt (the shape of the organisation as a whole). Organisational culture is accessed through immersion in the field rather than through the administration of a structured questionnaire.

Case studies

Much early organisational studies was based on case studies, and there has been a rediscovery of this tradition over the last twenty years. Methods typically include observation, semi-structured interviews and the analysis of documentary material. The objective is often to portray the organisation as a whole, or to trace how particular issues are processed or decisions taken. Organisations are followed up through time, which takes account of the impact of history. The handling of time and the creation of periods is then an important task, through conceptualising characteristic rates or patterns of organisational change (Weick and Quinn 1999). Cases may be analytic descriptions, where empirical material is both presented and then analysed against wider models or theories.

An important distinction is between single-case ethnographies (Box 2.3) and other case study designs. The exemplar case is used in much management teaching (the Harvard case study method) whereby students are expected to diagnose the key management problem in the text presented. This provides teaching material for students who wish to work in the management consultancy sector, and the cases frequently exhibit an action bias. While academic researchers criticise this approach, some influential and high-quality management texts (Argyris 1999) are derived from such reflections on consultancy work undertaken with leading companies.

A third approach is where the aim is to develop or test theory. Such explanatory case studies may be seen by some as examples of high-quality work within organisational studies. For example, Blau (1955) tried to operationalise the Weberian ideal type of a bureaucracy within two government agencies. Kanter's classic organisational study, *Men and Women of the Corporation*, worked to the following objective: 'the study represents primarily a search for explanation and theory rather than just a report of an empirical research' (Kanter 1977).

Researchers may operationalise wider social science concepts, testing them within particular organisational settings. For example, Harrison and colleagues' exploration of the impact of general management in the British NHS (1992) used the concepts of power and culture as organising devices. Inductive methods can be used whereby concepts emerge through carefully selected comparative case study data, as in an analysis of the capacity of health care organisations to progress strategic change (Pettigrew *et al.* 1992). This raises the question of pattern recognition within multiple cases where recent methodological guidance is available (Langley 1999). The view proposed here is that the use of multiple case studies which leads to the development of theory may be seen as a prime way forward in producing 'well conducted' organisational studies (Bowns and McNulty 1999) (Box 2.4).

Box 2.4 'Boys in white'

This is a case study from the Chicago School of the ideological and institutional role of one American medical school.

The researchers were interested in whether the medical school acted as a 'total institution' that not only imparted a body of knowledge but also socialised students into a particular culture. Although the unit of analysis was one organisation, there was a sophisticated sampling strategy for selecting a range of student groups within the organisation, so that there was multiple case analysis within the single case (see also Bowns and McNulty 1999 for a recent British example of this strategy).

The researchers undertook prolonged periods of observation of particular student groups, noting and recording key interactions and phrases within detailed fieldwork notes. These data were exhaustively coded and subjected to simple counting. They also used some questionnaires to supplement observational work.

This work is notable for an excellent 'Methods' chapter which operationalises the principles of grounded theory. The work also clearly relates the empirical data to wider theories about total institutions and the reproduction of occupational cultures.

(Becker *et al.* 1961)

Text as data

'Texts' created by organisations are analysed by postmodernist and poststructuralist scholars (Stablien 1996). Such scholars deny the existence of any reality other than the text itself as representative of a specific perspective at that point in time. As presented by the original author, the text constitutes a reality, which can then be deconstructed through textual analysis into multiple meanings. Not every text provides data for deconstruction – the most useful are those which are influential, so-called foundational texts.

The linguistic analysis of texts (such as annual reports or plans) may provide clues to persuasion devices and the emergence of new ideological positions and discourses. Such analysis might include a simple counting of the number of times a key word (such as 'enterprise' or 'leadership') appears or, more interestingly, a qualitative exploration of the relationship between words or phrases within the text.

Organisational action research

Action research represents an important development in research methods as a whole, implying a different relationship between research and practice than is evident within biomedical research or even conventional organisational studies (see Chapter 11). Much action research has taken place within an organisational context (Reason 1994), designed to facilitate organisational learning and change, possibly linked to consultancy interventions.

The question arises as to whether organisational action research can be seen as rigorous in research terms. Can it contribute to theory or systemic learning as well as local practice development? The work of Chris Argyris (1999) and his use of so-called Action Science to promote organisational learning involves using material generated in management development workshops to illustrate generic patterns of organisational and individual learning. Detailed notes are taken of particular interventions or conversations and subjected to exhaustive coding. On the basis of this material, a dominant organisational learning style can be deduced. This work clearly contributes to general concepts or theories (such as the existence of different learning styles) as well as localised learning for practice. Eden and Huxham (1996) also argue that action research can be used to promote the development of theory, albeit of an emergent and practice-relevant nature. Such theory is likely to be substantive (that is, lower-level and related to particular settings) in nature rather than general (that is, higher-level, abstracted, or axiomatic). These issues are considered further in Chapter 11.

Generalisation and overviews

Some organisational researchers are concerned by the need to ensure study replication and so promote generalisability (Donaldson 1996). Critics argue that the results of ethnography or single case studies are too localised to provide a secure base for policy. The replication of studies within different time periods or geographic sites is one way of establishing the extent to which generalisations can be safely made. For those researchers who wish to maintain a dialogue with policy makers, providing overviews across small clusters of related studies which have adopted similar methods is another approach to 'scaling up'.

Within organisational studies, the search for generalisability across completed research studies is often handled through personal overviews rather than the systematic reviews characteristic of health technology assessment (see Chapter 12). For example, Donaldson (1996) has reviewed thirty-five contingency theoretic studies, all of which came to similar conclusions, even within dissimilar national cultures. Nevertheless, some single case studies have had a major influence on the scholarly and indeed the policy world (Goffman 1961).

Limitations of organisational studies

So what are the limitations of organisational studies specifically within health care? It is weak on modelling the relationships between inputs and outcomes and strong on questions of intermediate process: an organisational study on the efficacy of aspirin in reducing the risk of heart attacks would be unlikely to produce valuable results. Its concern is typically for how systems evolve over time rather than establishing causality.

It is not good at studying the dynamics of individuals or small teams, where social psychologists have more expertise. It also sees the world through a presumption of strong social relations, and may not be useful where such relations are disintegrating, or where there is an increase in *anomie* (or normlessness) or the emergence of sharp market forces that overwhelm embedded social relations. Criticisms from health economists typically argue that organisational studies over-emphasise the restraining effects of culture or institutions and underplay the role of incentives in provoking novel forms of social action: organisational scholars see human beings as over-socialised and as unable to choose.

Organisational studies should be seen as an academic form of research, and requires longer timescales than would be expected from management consultancies or highly developmental approaches.

Like many social sciences, organisational studies is highly contestable (Reed 1996), with important internal debates. There is a lack of consensus (Tranfield and Starkey 1998), with no universally agreed methodological paradigm or theoretical stance. The subject is, rather, characterised by many different theoretical stances which remain in dispute, and by a range of methods. It does not display the equivalent of a 'hierarchy of evidence' model which can be used to order data (see Chapter 12). Often empirical findings are small-scale or not cumulative, and the craft of aggregating across projects is primitive. While empirical findings are important, such studies are unlikely to provide clear, unambiguous answers, and may require a process of intensive dialogue with policy makers to secure influence or acceptance (as propounded in Pawson and Tilley's 1997 account of the highly interactive nature of the interface between policy and research).

Organisational studies needs to be complemented by organisational economics (see Chapter 8) which has alternative theories (such as transaction costs theory) and socio-legal studies (such as contracting theory). Disciplines such as anthropology also provide useful expertise in such areas as ethnography and the exploration of organisational cultures.

The interface between organisational studies and the policy system may produce difficulties. On the one hand, organisational studies exhibits an applied component, with many researchers concerned to produce findings – and to undertake empirical studies – which are of interest to practitioners. On the other hand, it lacks a clear, shared purpose or measurement system. These 'soft' and 'divergent' characteristics of organisational studies (Tranfield and Starkey 1998) suggest that it is unlikely to produce universally agreed findings within a quick timescale: almost any findings are indeed likely to be subject to critique and debate from different subgroups of researchers.

Some organisational theory has been developed within the context of private sector firms (e.g. Porter's [1980] model of strategy under conditions of competition). Some private sector based models can be usefully applied within public sector organisations, as long as due attention is paid to the need to customise and adapt them where appropriate (Ferlie 2001). Other models, including Porter's, which assume the operation of competitive markets, are restricted in their public sector applicability. Yet other models which are broader in scope can apply to organisations in either sector (such as the resource-based view of the firm). Many early organisational studies were conducted within public sector settings, and such work has contributed to general theory (such as Mintzberg's [1979] model of a professionalised bureaucracy, based on his work in hospitals) rather than health care specific theory. The growth of the language of strategic management within contemporary public sector organisations is an example of an increased use of generic management concepts, within health care.

Further reading

Brock, D., Powell, M. and Hinings, C. R. (1999) *Restructuring The Professional Organisation*, London: Routledge.

Bryman, A. (1992) *Research Methods and Organisational Studies*, London: Routledge.

Clegg, S., Hardy, C. and Nord, W. (eds) (1996) *Handbook of Organisational Studies*, London: Sage.

Goffman, E. (1961) *Asylums*, London: Penguin.

Harrison, S., Hunter, D., Marnoch, G. and Pollitt, C. (1992) *Just Managing: Power and Culture in the NHS*, London: Macmillan.

Mabey, C. and Mayon-White, B. (1993) *Managing Change*, London: Paul Chapman Publishing.

Pettigrew, A., Ferlie, E. and McKee, L. (1992) *Managing Strategic Change*, London: Sage.

Shortell, S., Gillies, R., Anderson, D., Erickson, K. M. and Mitchell, J. B. (1996) *Remaking Health Care in America*, San Francisco: Jossey-Bass.

Starkey, K. (ed.) (1996) *How Organisations Learn*, London: International Thomson Business Press.

References

Aiken, M. and Hage, J. (1971) 'The organic organisation and innovation', *Sociology*, 5: 63–81.

Argyris, C. (1999) *On Organisational Learning*, Oxford: Blackwell.

Becker, H., Geer, B., Hughes, E. and Strauss, A. (1961) *Boys in White*, Chicago: University of Chicago Press.

Blau, P. (1955) *The Dynamics of Bureaucracy*, Chicago: University of Chicago Press.

Bowns, I. and McNulty, T. (1999) *Reengineering LRI: An Independent Evaluation of Implementation and Impact*, Sheffield: SCHARR/CCSC, University of Sheffield.

Brock, D., Powell, M. and Hinings, C. R. (1999) *Restructuring the Professional Organisation*, London: Routledge.

Bryman, A. (1992) *Research Methods and Organisational Studies*, London: Routledge.

Campbell, D. T. and Stanley, J. C. (1966) *Experimental and Quasi Experimental Designs for Research*, Chicago: Rand McNally.

Clegg, S., Hardy, C. and Nord, W. (eds) (1996) *Handbook of Organisational Studies*, London: Sage.

Cooke, B. (1999) 'Writing the Left out of management theory – the historiography of the management of change', *Organisation*, 6, 1: 81–105.

Davies, B. P. and Challis, D. (1986) *Matching Resources to Needs in Community Care*, Aldershot: Gower.

Denzin, N. and Lincoln, Y. (1994) *Handbook of Qualitative Research*, London: Sage.

Donaldson, L. (1996) 'The normal science of structural contingency theory', in S. Clegg, C. Hardy and W. Nord (eds) *Handbook of Organisational Studies*, 57–76, London: Sage.

Eden, C. and Huxham, C. (1996) 'Action research for the study of organisations', in S. Clegg, C. Hardy and W. Nord (eds) *Handbook of Organisational Studies*, 526–42, London: Sage.

Ferlie, E. (2001) 'Quasi strategy: strategic management in the contemporary public sector', in A. Pettigrew, H. Thomas and R. Whittington (eds) *Sage Handbook of Strategy and Management*, London: Sage, in press.

Ferlie, E., Ashburner, L., FitzGerald, L. and Pettigrew, A. (1996) *The New Public Management in Action*, Oxford: Oxford University Press.

Goffman, E. (1961) *Asylums*, London: Penguin.

Harrison, S., Hunter, D., Marnoch, G. and Pollitt, C. (1992) *Just Managing: Power and Culture in the NHS*, London: Macmillan.

Joss, R. and Kogan, M. (1995) *Advancing Quality*, Buckingham: Open University Press.

Kanter, R. M. (1977) *Men and Women of the Corporation*, New York: Basic Books.

Langley, A. (1999) 'Strategies for theorising from process data', *Academy of Management Review*, 24, 4: 691–710.

Lewin, K. (1951) *Field Theory in Social Science*, New York: HarperCollins.

Mark, A. and Dopson, S. (1999) *Organisational Behaviour in Health Care*, London: Macmillan.

Mintzberg, H. (1979) *The Structuring of Organisations*, Englewood Cliffs NJ: Prentice Hall.

Pawson, R. and Tilley, N. (1997) *Realistic Evaluation*, London: Sage.

Peters, T. J. and Waterman, R. (1982) *In Search of Excellence*, New York: Harper and Row.

Pettigrew, A., Ferlie, E. and McKee, L. (1992) *Managing Strategic Change*, London: Sage.

Porter, M. (1980) *Competitive Strategy*, New York: Free Press.

Pugh, D. (1997) 'Does context determine form?', in D. Pugh (ed.) *Organisation Theory: Selected Readings*, London: Penguin.

Reason, P. (1994) 'Three approaches to participative enquiry', in N. Denzin and Y. Lincoln (eds) *Handbook of Qualitative Research*, London: Sage.

Reed, M. (1996) 'Organisational theorising: a historically contested terrain', in S. Clegg, C. Hardy and W. Nord (eds) *Handbook of Organisational Studies*, 31–56, London: Sage.

Runciman, W. G. (ed.) (1978) *Weber: Selections in Translation*, Cambridge: Cambridge University Press.

Schein, E. (1985) *Organisational Culture and Leadership*, San Francisco: Jossey-Bass.

Senge, P. (1990) *The Fifth Discipline*, London: Century Business.

Shortell, S., Jones, R., Rademaker, A., Gillies, R., Dranove, D., Hughes, E., Budetti, P., Reynolds, K. and Huang, C. (2000) 'Assessing the impact of TQM and organisational culture on multiple outcomes for care for coronary artery bypass graft surgery patients', *Medical Care*, 38, 2: 207–17.

Stablein, R. (1996) 'Data in organisation studies', in S. Clegg, C. Hardy and W. Nord (eds) *Handbook of Organisational Studies*, 509–25, London: Sage.

Strauss, A., Schatzman, L. Bucher, R., Elrich, D. and Sabstin, M. (1964) *Psychiatric Ideologies and Institutions*, London: Collier Macmillan.

Tranfield, D. and Starkey, K. (1998) 'The nature, social organisation and promotion of management research: towards policy', *British Journal of Management*, 9: 341–53.

Weick, K. and Quinn, R. (1999) 'Organisational change and development', *Annual Review of Psychology*, 50: 361–86.

Woodward, J. (1965) *Industrial Organisation*, Oxford: Oxford University Press.

Chapter 3

Micro-level qualitative research

Elizabeth Murphy

Introduction

The legitimacy and usefulness of the contribution of qualitative research to studying the organisation and delivery of health services are hotly contested. Enthusiasts argue that qualitative research has an essential contribution to make to the study of health care settings, while critics respond that such methods lack rigour and precision. This debate is, at times, vituperative, with qualitative researchers condemning alternative approaches as scientistic, positivistic, artificial and failing to reflect meanings underpinning social action. Critics are equally outspoken, rejecting qualitative research as soft, impressionistic, anecdotal, political and subjective. On both sides there is a tendency to present qualitative methods as innovative, controversial and relatively untried. In fact, self-conscious discussion of qualitative methods in social research has been around for at least one hundred years (Dingwall *et al.* 1998) and the terms in which the current debate is conducted are anticipated in much earlier writings on the subject (Murphy *et al.* 1998).

This chapter focuses on researching health service delivery and organisation issues at the micro level, i.e. below the level of the organisation, contrasting with Chapter 2 of this volume, where methods for studying these issues at the level of the organisation are discussed, and with Chapter 6 where macro considerations dominate. It begins by outlining some of the dimensions of contemporary debates about the nature and purpose of qualitative research, suggesting the limitations of some of those positions outlined for research into the delivery and organisation of health care. It then considers some types of research question for which qualitative research methods may be particularly appropriate, before going on to outline the principal methods adopted by qualitative researchers, illustrating these with examples drawn from the health field.

Definition and theoretical basis

Arguments about the usefulness of qualitative methods are dogged by the lack of consensus, among advocates as much as among opponents, about both the definition and the purpose of qualitative research. Initially, the definition of qualitative research appears relatively unproblematic. Qualitative research deals with data not easily reduced to numbers. It focuses on questions such as, 'What is going on here?' and 'How does this come to happen in this setting?', rather than asking 'How much?', 'How often?' and 'How many?'. This is not to suggest that qualitative researchers never engage in counting exercises (Silverman 1985), but rather that production and manipulation of numerical data are not the central goal of the research. By this definition, qualitative research would include observational studies of naturally occurring interactions in health care settings, analysis of audio or video recordings of such interactions, non-standardised individual and group interviews with providers and recipients of health care, and the analysis of documentary material produced in health care settings. At this level, the debate about qualitative research concerns the appropriateness of certain methods for studying the delivery and organisation of health services. The question we need to ask about such methods is whether they are well suited to answering some of the questions that arise at the micro level.

Before doing so, however, we should recognise that the debate about qualitative methods is complicated by cross-cutting arguments about methodology (see Chapter 1). There is a marked lack of consensus within the qualitative research community about the ontology and epistemology of their work, and any debate about the usefulness of such research is confounded by claims about which philosophical assumptions are or are not central to qualitative and/or quantitative research.

Some argue that qualitative and quantitative research are founded upon fundamentally different and inescapably opposed philosophical assumptions. The distinction between the two is said to be both ontological and epistemological (Smith 1983). This is linked to the assertion that qualitative and quantitative research are grounded in different and opposing paradigms (Smith and Heshusius 1986; Dootson 1995) (see Chapters 1 and 2). A paradigm is 'the basic belief system or world view that guides the investigator, not only in choices of method but in ontologically and epistemologically fundamental ways' (Guba and Lincoln 1994: 105). Qualitative research is represented as an 'alternative paradigm'. At times the term paradigm is used somewhat loosely, simply to suggest that qualitative and quantitative researchers stress different priorities. However, some influential qualitative researchers go much further than this, arguing that qualitative and quantitative research are different paradigms in the full sense of the word outlined above.

Guba and Lincoln argue that decisions about paradigms should take precedence over decisions about methods (Guba and Lincoln 1994; Lincoln and Guba 2000). While Lincoln (1990) identifies qualitative methods as central to the alternative or constructivist paradigm she advocates, she allows that in some circumstances quantitative methods might justifiably be employed if they conform to alternative paradigm assumptions. There is for Lincoln and Guba, however, no possibility of legitimately combining paradigms. Given the radical disjunction between the assumptions of this 'alternative' paradigm and those underpinning conventional approaches within health services approaches, this effectively rules out combining qualitative methods with most health services research as currently practised.

What characterises this 'alternative paradigm' which its advocates link so closely to qualitative research? Most fundamentally, it is associated with a rejection of the realist assumption that 'the world has an existence independent of our perception of it' (Williams and May 1996: 81). Consequently, it is associated with a commitment to ontological idealism and epistemological relativism. Idealism involves the rejection of the notion that reality exists 'out there' or can be known 'objectively'. In other words, what we take to be reality is created (or, in some versions of idealism, shaped) by our minds.

The implications of adopting either a realist or an idealist position become clear when we turn to the notions of 'validity' and 'truth' implied by the two positions. For realists, findings are valid if they correspond to external reality (Hammersley 1992). Idealism rejects correspondence with reality as an appropriate goal. From this perspective, it is possible for many, even contradictory, truths to exist alongside one another (Guba and Lincoln 1989). Thus idealism is closely associated with relativism. A researcher's account is just one version of the world among others. Guba and Lincoln observe (1989: 86, original italics): 'It is dubious that the constructivist paradigm requires a term like *truth*, which has a final or ultimate ring to it'.

The potentially negative consequences of a radically relativist position for policy-oriented research have been identified (Schwandt 1997; Atkinson and Hammersley 1994; Campbell 1994; Hammersley 1992). If all that researchers can hope to do is to spawn multiple, incommensurable, potentially contradictory versions of the world, on the basis of the same research experience, it is difficult to justify the expenditure of public money on such research. This position denies us critical purchase on members' accounts, be they professionals, managers, patients or carers (Schwandt 1997).

Is Smith (1983) right to suggest that qualitative research is inextricably bound up with radical idealist assumptions? I think not. These are *a priori* assumptions, which are not open to scientific investigation or refutation. In practice, not all qualitative research is associated with idealist assumptions. Indeed, Hammersley and Atkinson (1995) have observed a tension at the heart of much qualitative research, with researchers juggling a realist position in relation to their own research reports while still treating the beliefs and perspectives of those they study as incommensurable, socially constructed accounts.

How then are we to choose between the various methodological positions on offer for studying the delivery and organisation of health services? I suggest that two appropriate grounds for such a choice are utility on the one hand and coherence on the other. As we have seen, the usefulness of policy-oriented research grounded in radical idealist and relativist assumptions is seriously compromised. However, this is not to say that realism (at least in its naive forms) offers a coherent alternative. Realist researchers who claim to uncover some aspect of objective reality fail to recognise that their observations are never purely the reflection of an external world. There is no possibility of 'theory-free' knowledge. All observations are theory-laden, and no degree of methodological sophistication will allow us to escape from this bind (Smith and Dresner 2000). This applies not only to the researcher's own observations but also to the accounts of members of the setting under study. One may reject the idealist position that many realities exist, and still hold firm to the important insight that different people observing the same reality may produce different versions of that reality.

This position, which Hammersley (1992) calls 'subtle realism', accepts that we cannot escape the social world in order to study it. Subtle realists maintain that reality does exist independently of the researcher's claims about it and that those claims may be more or less accurate. They concede that it is never possible to make knowledge claims if we cannot be fully certain of their validity. Rather, our search should be for knowledge about whose accuracy we can be reasonably confident. Here validity becomes a 'regulative ideal' (Phillips 1987: 23). Very importantly, subtle realists distance themselves from the goal of *reproducing* reality. Rather, they seek to *represent* reality, recognising that phenomena can be represented from different perspectives. Each perspective is potentially true. Thus multiple, *non-competing*, complementary valid descriptions are possible. What are not possible, for the subtle realist, are multiple, *contradictory*, valid descriptions of the kind for which idealists argue.

Subtle realism represents an appropriate methodological foundation for qualitative (and indeed quantitative) research into health service delivery and organisation. It avoids the polarities of both radical idealism and radical realism. It allows us to incorporate elements of social constructionism and a recognition of the impact of culture upon observation, without abandoning the search for independent knowledge about health care delivery and organisation. It undermines the claim that qualitative research is grounded in an alternative paradigm, and removes barriers to creative combinations of qualitative and quantitative research.

Uses of micro-level qualitative research

Qualitative methods may be used to study settings that are inaccessible to other research methods. These might include, for example, genito-urinary clinics or drug treatment and other facilities catering for people engaged in stigmatised or illegal activities. Other examples of settings difficult to access are those, such as palliative care units, where interactions are likely to be highly sensitive. In all these examples, carrying out sample surveys or intervention studies might pose significant practical and ethical difficulties.

Qualitative methods also provide a rigorous descriptive base for subsequent research or to provide policy makers and practitioners with a sound knowledge of the contexts for implementing new policies or practices. A feature of routine work is that professionals cease to notice the mundane aspects of their practice and how such practice is constrained by the settings in which it is carried out. Similarly, they may fail to observe the impact their own practices have upon others in the setting. Qualitative research can be a powerful tool in identifying such 'seen but unnoticed' (Garfinkel 1967: 36) aspects of settings and interactions.

In particular, qualitative research is well suited to studying the processual and dynamic nature of the phenomena under study. As such, it can complement the findings of input/output studies. As Dingwall (1992) argued, input/output (or 'black box') studies fail to provide some of the information that is required by policy makers and planners. Such studies can establish the presence or absence of a link between an input and an output: however, they are not able to establish the process through which the input has led to the output. This is a particular problem, given the high degree of 'local customisation' to which, in practice, health care interventions are subject (see Chapter 2). Qualitative research and, in particular, observational studies offer one means by which such processes can be documented.

Furthermore, qualitative research can contribute to refining concepts and generating hypotheses for subsequent research. This may help to avoid 'grapeshot' research, where one measures all possible variables, hoping some turn out to be significant. It can prevent premature conceptualisation of variables and arbitrary selection of the relationships to be examined, and consequent waste of funds invested in quantitative research.

At the other end of the research cycle, qualitative research can help to interpret the findings of quantitative research. This is particularly so where quantitative research throws up unexpected findings or identifies exceptional cases that do not fit with the generality. Examining such exceptional cases using qualitative methods may allow us to refine further probabilistic rules inferred from the analysis of quantitative data.

Qualitative methods also play an important role in enhancing the generalisability of intervention studies. Having established the usefulness of an innovation in a study setting, one cannot be sure it will be equally useful in other settings. One reason for this is that, particularly in service delivery, one is always dealing with an interaction between innovation and context. A distinctive feature of qualitative research is a concern with studying the phenomenon of interest in context. Careful presentation, based on rigorous qualitative data analysis, of the context in which an innovation took place, can facilitate application of findings beyond study settings.

Finally, people's behaviour in interactions is influenced by their beliefs as well as by 'objective' reality. Resisting the temptation to 'fix meanings' is central to qualitative research. Qualitative researchers seek to infer meanings underpinning action by observing action in context. This is particularly useful in identifying factors that sustain professional or patient practices that are demonstrably either inappropriate or harmful.

How to undertake micro-level qualitative research

Qualitative research incorporates various methods of data collection and analysis that may be used separately or in combination. These include direct observation of naturally occurring events and behaviour (participant or non-participant observation), fine-grained analysis of audio or video recordings of interactions (interaction analysis), qualitative individual and group interviews, and the analysis of documentary material.

Participant or non-participant observation

Here an individual researcher or members of a research team engage in the daily life of the group or setting under study. They watch, listen and record what happens in the everyday interactions, involving themselves to a greater (participant) or lesser (non-participant) extent in ongoing activities (Box 3.1). Typically, the observation period is lengthy, often six months or more. The number of settings is small and, in many cases, only one setting is

---

Box 3.1 Non-participant observational study of how neonatal intensive care works

This study of neonatal intensive care is a good example of an observational study of health care delivery at the micro level. The researchers identified their goal as a 'dispassionate assessment of how the system works'. Their principal research setting was a neonatal unit in the eastern United States. For six months they attended weekly discussions of problem cases with nurses, social workers, doctors and other consulting professionals. They then began an eight-month observation period, spending extended periods in the unit. Following observations in this primary site, they visited fourteen other regional units in the USA and comparable units in England, the Netherlands, East and West Germany, France and Brazil. These shorter visits gave a perspective on national and international variations in the delivery and organisation of neonatal intensive care.

Having developed a sound descriptive base from their observational data, they identified policy and practice issues raised by the study. They highlighted the huge expansion of neonatal intensive care without specific and uniform policies that emphasised the needs of newborn infants. They noted a lack of clear and publicly endorsed agreement about appropriate and equitable selection of patients, the extent to which social factors and parental wishes could legitimately be taken into account in treatment decisions, and about when treatment could and should be instigated and sustained. They detailed the complex process of decision making in the units, and the way external bureaucratic imperatives impinged upon treatment decisions. They described the role played by different professional groups, the influence these had upon treatment decisions, and how treatment dilemmas were negotiated and resolved. They studied interactions between parents and professionals, and how professionals managed parents.

Recommendations from this study addressed three levels of decision making – the unit, the hospital and the government. At the unit level, the study reported that the initiation of aggressive, heroic interventions was often routine, even when the baby was clearly dying. They observed that this resulted partly from a lack of procedures for evaluating the babies after admission. They advocated making formal re-evaluation of the benefits versus the detriments of treatment for each baby as standard practice twenty-four hours after admission.

(Guillemin and Holmstrom 1986)

studied. Increasingly, however, researchers combine intensive study of one setting with shorter observations at additional sites in an attempt to extend the generalisability of findings from the principal setting.

Data analysis is based upon detailed field notes. In making such notes, the objective is to provide a comprehensive record of what is observed in a setting. Ideally, verbal interactions are recorded verbatim. In the early stages, researchers familiarise themselves with the setting, but as time goes on observations become more focused. Hypotheses generated in the early stages are tested in the later stages. The researcher seeks out cases or incidents that challenge, contradict or refine early observations. Analysis is ongoing throughout the study, rather than being concentrated at the end.

Interaction analysis

In this refinement of observation, the researcher uses audio or video recording to examine interactions in fine detail. It is particularly useful where the phenomenon of interest is contained in fairly static settings, permitting unobtrusive recording (Box 3.2). Much health care occurs in such settings. Recorded data are transcribed, using detailed notation that retains

---

Box 3.2 Interaction analysis of the impact of computerisation on general practice

The researchers video-recorded consultations before and after the installation of a computer system in an inner-city general practice in north-west England. The recordings were played repeatedly and carefully transcribed. The researchers transcribed not only what was said, but also details of speech production, including pauses, overlaps, non-verbal utterances, changes in pitch and amplitude, audible inhalations, and so on. Visual conduct, such as gaze direction and gesture, was also transcribed. Approximately 100 pre-installation and 150 post-installation consultations with seven GPs were recorded. The installation of computers was found to undermine significantly doctors' ability to document and retrieve information while, at the same time, displaying sensitivity to the needs of the patient. The researchers identified design features of the particular computer system being used which exacerbated this difficulty, and ways in which GPs could retain the system but minimise the impact upon interactions with patients.

(Greatbatch et al. 1995)

---

not only words spoken but also pauses, intonation, overlapping talk, non-verbal contributions and so on. This attention to fine detail allows the researcher to analyse tacit, 'seen but unnoticed' background features of interactions. This approach has been used widely to study the structuring of talk within medical consultations.

Interviews

Qualitative interviews with individuals and groups are widely used in studies at the micro level. Such interviews are often seen as offering the patient perspective on care, or identifying features of the patient's understanding that influence response to treatment. The adoption of qualitative interview techniques can be understood as a reaction against highly standardised interviews, which are criticised for imposing the researcher's categories and priorities and, in the process, distorting the respondent's understanding.

Qualitative interviews vary in their degree of structure. Sometimes the researcher works from an interview guide which specifies topics to be covered, possibly with a range of questions and prompts. This interview guide may be used flexibly, allowing informants to discuss topics in any order and to propose new areas of relevance. In less structured interviews, respondents may simply be invited to talk about an area, in whatever way they choose, with minimal interviewer direction. Such interviews are usually mechanically recorded, transcribed, and then subject to detailed analysis. Data are coded, often with codes developed during the analysis.

A number of advantages are claimed for qualitative interviews, some of which are highly contentious. Such interviews are frequently presented as giving access to informants' own definitions of their experiences and practices (e.g. Secker *et al.* 1995). It is claimed that they allow the informant to 'tell it how it is', whether 'it' is the experience of having cancer therapy, antenatal care, or whatever. Unlike standardised interviews, qualitative interviews are held to avoid the pitfall of imposing researcher assumptions on informants, and to allow informants to define what is significant or important.

There is some truth in such claims. Qualitative interviews can certainly highlight dimensions that the researcher has overlooked, fulfilling a useful 'hypothesis generating' function. They can encourage researchers to recognise the legitimacy of cultural differences between informants' accounts and their own. At times, however, this argument shades over into a claim that qualitative interviews allow us to penetrate the informant's mental world and to discover what they *really* think about the phenomenon of interest. As a result, it is argued, such interviews allow us to extract a 'truer' version of events or experiences than is allowed when using more structured methods.

This claim that qualitative interviews offer us access to a more valid version of reality than is possible using standardised techniques has been subject to a mounting challenge since the publication of Cicourel's book *Method and Measurement* (1964), in 1964 (Dingwall 1997). All interviews, whether qualitative or quantitative, are contextually situated social interactions. As such they are inevitably occasions for 'impression management' (Goffman 1959) on which both interviewers and informants seek to present themselves as competent and sane members of their community (Dingwall 1997). This means that we cannot treat informants' talk as reproducing their mental states, opinions, understandings or preferences. Rather, such interview talk is social action, and this has potentially radical implications for the analysis of interview talk (Box 3.3).

Box 3.3 Non-participant observation and interviews: delivery of care in British general practice

The researchers studied two general practices in a South Wales town. They used a combination of methods, including direct observation of consultations, individual and group interviews with patients, and informal conversations with practice staff. In analysing their data, they noticed marked inconsistencies between the behaviour observed in consultations and the interview accounts patients offered of such consultations. In the observations, the patients were almost invariably passive and appeared reluctant to challenge or question their doctors. However, patients' interview accounts of consultations took the form of dramatic presentations with the patient cast as hero and the doctor as incompetent. In contrast to the observational data, patients presented themselves as active and the doctors as passive. The stories patients told about their medical encounters were a 'vehicle for making the patient appear rational and sensible and for redressing imbalance between patient and doctor'.

(Stimson and Webb 1975)

The discrepancies between observational and interview data certainly appear to undermine the usefulness of interview data as literal reports of reality. However, this does not mean that interviews are fundamentally flawed as sources of evidence. The central lesson is not so much about data collection as about analysis. It is necessary to analyse interview data in terms of what respondents are *doing* with their talk. This approach to interview data, rather than judging whether interviewees' accounts are 'true', reflects on and attempts to understand the 'situated work' (Dingwall 1981) that they do. This perspective on interview accounts has considerable potential for informing the delivery of health care (Box 3.4).

Box 3.4 A study of parents of children attending a clinic for congenital heart disease

Baruch interviewed thirty-two families, inviting parents to 'tell the story' of their child's 'career' in the hospital clinic. A striking feature of these interviews was the telling of 'atrocity stories' about dysfunctional encounters with health professionals. Like Stimson and Webb (see Box 3.3), Baruch resisted the temptation to analyse these stories as more or less accurate reproductions of the incompetence or insensitivity of professionals. Rather, he examined parents' accounts for what they revealed about being a parent in such health care settings. He noted how the structure and organisation of the clinics served to undermine parents' construction of themselves as adequate parents and the way this occasioned the kinds of moral repair work the parents engaged in as they told atrocity stories. His analysis led to the introduction of an additional clinic session in which parents could ask questions and 'engage in a display of parental responsibility'.

(Baruch 1981; Silverman 1985: 175)

Studies such as these require us to exercise some caution in interpreting the data from patient satisfaction studies. Where such studies rely upon self-reported satisfaction, we would do well to consider not only what patients say but also what they are doing as they say it.

Documents

Health care settings produce large amounts of documentary data: patient records, referral and discharge letters, test results, treatment plans, case reports, patient information leaflets and so on. In addition to naturally occurring documents, researchers also commission documentary materials such as diaries and journals. As with interview data, the status given to documentary data varies between qualitative research traditions. Finnegan (1996) distinguishes between those who make direct and indirect use of documents.

Direct use treats documents as at least potentially accurate sources of information. For example, one might analyse hospital personnel records for information about the mobility of nursing staff between different specialities within the hospital.

Indirect use of documentary material involves analysing documents in terms of what they reveal about the perspectives and priorities of different members within settings. Here, documents are treated as contextually produced.

Limitations of micro-level qualitative research

Qualitative research at the micro level is well suited to answering some questions about the delivery and organisation of health care. It is rarely an appropriate or cost-effective response where the objective is to establish the extent or frequency of phenomena.

Qualitative research is highly labour-intensive and, unlike some other methods of data collection and analysis, demands the highest level of expertise to undertake the 'hands-on' research. This is different from, for example, survey research, where as long as the experts set the study and analysis up well and give clear instructions, it is possible to delegate much data collection and analysis. In qualitative research, the emergent nature of data collection and analysis demands greater day-to-day, hands-on involvement from project directors – a level of involvement that is often difficult to reconcile with other responsibilities and commitments.

Perhaps the most frequently discussed reservation about qualitative research relates to the generalisability of its findings. Qualitative research is frequently accused of anecdotalism and hence of being of little practical use to policy makers and practitioners. In some cases, of course, the generalisation of findings is immaterial. This might apply, for example, where the research objective is the evaluation of an innovation in a single setting, where there is no intention to replicate the programme in other contexts. In most cases, however, the usefulness of research is enhanced when its findings can be taken to inform our understanding of contexts or individuals beyond those who are the subject of a particular study. The justification for funding research into the delivery and organisation of health care is generally less in terms of the uniqueness of a particular individual or setting than of the extent to which findings from such cases can be extrapolated to other similar cases.

There are those who reject generalisability as an appropriate goal within qualitative research (Stake 1995). At the extreme, attempts to generalise across social settings have been described as an act of despotism (Lyotard 1993). Others take a more moderate view but are nevertheless concerned that preoccupation with generalisation may have a distorting effect upon research. It may distract the researcher from what Stake sees as the primary goal of a qualitative case study, that of offering the reader vicarious experience of an individual case. The uniqueness of every research setting and particular characteristics of qualitative methods (e.g. theoretical sampling, emergent design, the large volume of data) are seen as major barriers to generalising findings beyond the particular setting studied (Duffy 1985).

It is certainly true that it is rarely practical in qualitative research to adopt the probabilistic sampling methods which are the basis of claims to generalisability in much quantitative research. While there are no principled objections to probability sampling in qualitative research (Hammersley 1992; LeCompte and Preissle 1993), the ratio of settings studied to the population to which one wishes to generalise is usually too low to permit statistical extrapolation. However, researchers can enhance the generalisability of their findings by making thoughtful sampling decisions, informed by evidence about the aggregate from which the sample is to be drawn. Such evidence may come from published statistics and/or original quantitative data collection (Hammersley 1992). In conducting the study, qualitative researchers may be able to strengthen their claim to generalisability by combining the intensive study of one or more cases with more targeted examination of a larger number of cases, to discover whether the observations made in the initial case(s) hold elsewhere (see Box 3.1).

Seale (1999) argues that readers of research reports must make their own decisions about the applicability of research findings to other contexts. Here, the location of the case studied within a theoretical framework is vital (see Chapter 2 in this volume). This may entail using research to test theories generated in other research, or generating theory from the data (e.g. Glaser and Strauss 1967) or, in some cases, a combination of both (Murphy *et al.* 1998). In addition, the potential for generalisability of findings will be enhanced by the inclusion in research reports of detailed descriptions of the context in which the research was carried out. Detailed descriptions (sometimes referred to as 'thick' descriptions) allow the reader to make an informed judgement about whether the similarities between the original setting and those to which the findings are to be applied are sufficient to give confidence that findings from one setting will hold in the others (Kennedy 1979).

Qualitative methods can contribute to cumulative knowledge about health service delivery and organisation in micro-level settings in a number of ways. The delivery and organisation of health care raise a wide range of research questions, some of which are amenable to investigation using qualitative methods while, for others, quantitative methods will be more appropriate. We are not faced with a stark choice between words and numbers in research (Hammersley 1992). Decisions about methods should be driven by a consideration of the purposes of the research, rather than prior ideological commitment to particular philosophical paradigms. Nor are those who use qualitative methods exempt from the standards of rigour that are reasonably expected from those who seek public money to undertake research. While it may never be possible to demonstrate the absolute validity of truth claims arising from any research, whether qualitative or quantitative, this does not relieve us of the responsibility to demonstrate that our findings are warranted, while recognising that truth may look somewhat different when viewed from different perspectives.

Acknowledgement

I am grateful to Robert Dingwall for comments on an earlier draft of this chapter.

Further reading

Bryman, A. (1988) *Quality and Quantity in Social Research*, London: Unwin Hyman.
Denzin, N. and Lincoln, Y. (2000) *Handbook of Qualitative Research*, London: Sage.
Hammersley, M. (1992) *What's Wrong with Ethnography?*, London: Routledge.
——(1995) *The Politics of Social Research*, London: Sage.
Hammersley, M. and Atkinson, P. (1993) *Ethnography: Principles in Practice*, 2nd edn, London: Routledge.
Miller, G. and Dingwall, R. (1997) *Context and Method in Qualitative Research*, London: Sage.
Murphy, E., Dingwall, R., Greatbatch, D., Parker, S. and Watson, P. (1998) 'Qualitative research methods in health technology assessment: a review of the literature', *Health Technology Assessment*, 2, 16: 1–276.
Seale, C. (1999) *The Quality of Qualitative Research*, London: Sage.
Silverman, D. (1993) *Interpreting Qualitative Data: Methods for Analysing Talk, Text and Interaction*, London: Sage.
——(2000) *Doing Qualitative Research*, London: Sage.

References

Atkinson, P. and Hammersley, M. (1994) 'Ethnography and participant observation', in N. Denzin and Y. Lincoln (eds) *Handbook of Qualitative Research*, 248–61, Thousand Oaks CA: Sage.
Baruch, G. (1981) 'Moral tales: parents' stories of encounters with the health profession', *Sociology of Health and Illness*, 3: 275–96.
Campbell, D. (1994) 'Can we overcome world-view incommensurability/relativity in trying to understand the other?', in R. Jessor, A. Colby and R. Shweder (eds) *Ethnography and Human Development: Context and Meaning in Social Inquiry*, 153–72, Chicago: University of Chicago Press.
Cicourel, A. V. (1964) *Method and Measurement in Sociology*, New York: Free Press.
Dingwall, R. (1981) 'The ethnomethodological movement', in G. Payne, R. Dingwall, J. Payne and M. Carter (eds) *Sociology and Social Research*, 124–38, London: Croom Helm.
——(1992) ' "Don't mind him – he's from Barcelona": qualitative methods in health studies', in J. Daly, I. McDonald and E. Wilks (eds) *Researching Health Care*, 161–7, London: Tavistock/Routledge.
——(1997) 'Accounts, interviews and observations', in G. Miller and R. Dingwall (eds) *Context and Method in Qualitative Research*, 51–65, London: Sage.
Dingwall, R., Murphy, E., Watson, P., Greatbatch, D. and Parker, S. (1998) 'Catching goldfish: quality in qualitative research', *Journal of Health Services Research & Policy*, 3, 3: 167–72.
Dootson, S. (1995) 'An in-depth study of triangulation', *Journal of Advanced Nursing*, 22, 183–7.
Duffy, M. (1985) 'Designing nursing research: the qualitative/quantitative debate', *Journal of Advanced Nursing*, 10, 225–32.
Finnegan, R. (1996) 'Using documents', in R. Sapsford and V. Jupp (eds) *Data Collection and Analysis*, 138–51, London: Sage.
Garfinkel, H. (1967) *Studies in Ethnomethodology*, Englewood Cliffs NJ: Prentice-Hall.

Glaser, B. G. and Strauss, A. L. (1967) *The Discovery of Grounded Theory: Strategies for Qualitative Research*, Chicago: Aldine.

Goffman, E. (1959) *The Presentation of Self in Everyday Life*, Harmondsworth: Penguin.

Greatbatch, D., Heath, C. C., Luff, P. and Campion, P. (1995) 'Conversation analysis: human/computer interaction and the general practice consultation', in A. Monk and N. Gilbert (eds) *Perspectives on Human/Computer Interaction*, 199–222, London: Academic Press.

Guba, E. G. and Lincoln, Y. S. (1989) *Fourth Generation Evaluation*, Newbury Park CA: Sage.

——(1994) 'Competing paradigms in qualitative research', in N. K. Denzin and Y. S. Lincoln (eds) *Handbook of Qualitative Research*, 105–17, Thousand Oaks CA: Sage.

Guillemin, J. H. and Holmstrom, L. L. (1986) *Mixed Blessings: Intensive Care For Newborns*, Oxford: Oxford University Press.

Hammersley, M. (1992) *What's Wrong with Ethnography?*, London: Routledge.

Hammersley, M. and Atkinson, P. (1995) *Ethnography: Principles in Practice*, London: Routledge.

Kennedy, M. (1979) 'Generalizing from single case studies', *Evaluation Quarterly*, 3: 661–78.

LeCompte, M. and Preissle, J. (1993) 'Selecting and sampling in qualitative research', in M. LeCompte and J. Preissle (eds) *Ethnography and Qualitative Design in Educational Research*, 2nd edn, 56–85, London: Academic Press.

Lincoln, Y. (1990) 'The making of a constructivist: a remembrance of transformations past', in E. Guba (ed.) *The Paradigm Dialog*, Newbury Park CA: Sage.

Lincoln, Y. and Guba, E. (2000) 'Paradigmatic controversies, contradictions, and emerging confluences', in N. Denzin and Y. Lincoln (eds) *Handbook of Qualitative Research*, 2nd edn, Thousand Oaks CA: Sage.

Lyotard, J. F. (1993) 'Answering the question: what is postmodernism?', in T. Docherty (ed.) *Postmodernism: A Reader*, 38–46, London: Harvester Wheatsheaf.

Murphy, E., Dingwall, R., Greatbatch, D., Parker, S. and Watson, P. (1998) 'Qualitative research methods in health technology assessment: a review of the literature', *Health Technology Assessment*, 2, 16: 1–276.

Phillips, D. (1987) 'Validity in qualitative research: why the worry about warrant will not wane', *Education and Urban Society*, 20: 9–24.

Schwandt, T. (1997) *Qualitative Inquiry: a Dictionary of Terms*, Thousand Oaks CA: Sage.

Seale, C. (1999) *The Quality of Qualitative Research*, London: Sage.

Secker, J., Wimbush, E., Watson, J. and Milburn, K. (1995) 'Qualitative methods in health promotion research: some criteria for quality', *Health Education Journal*, 54, 74–87.

Silverman, D. (1985) *Qualitative Methodology and Sociology*, 1st edn, Aldershot: Gower.

Smith, J. (1983) 'Quantitative versus interpretive: the problem of conducting social inquiry', in E. House (ed.) *Philosophy of Evaluation*, 27–51, San Francisco: Jossey-Bass.

Smith, J. and Heshusius, L. (1986) 'Closing down the conversation: the end of the quantitative/qualitative debate among educational inquirers', *Educational Researcher*, 15, 4–12.

Smith, J. K. and Dresner, D. K. (2000) 'The problem of criteria in the age of relativism', in N. Denzin and Y. Lincoln (eds) *Handbook of Qualitative Research*, 877–96, London: Sage.

Stake, R. (1995) *The Art of Case Study Research*, Thousand Oaks CA: Sage.

Stimson, G. and Webb, B. (1975) *Going to See the Doctor*, London: Routledge.

Williams, M. and May, T. (1996) *Introduction to the Philosophy of Social Research*, London: UCL Press.

Chapter 4

Epidemiological methods

Jeremy Grimshaw, Brenda Wilson, Marion Campbell, Martin Eccles and Craig Ramsay

Introduction

In this chapter we describe epidemiological approaches, focusing particularly on methods for estimating the magnitude of the benefits of interventions to improve the delivery and organisation of health services. This type of evaluation informs the choice of interventions or policies by identifying and estimating the advantages and disadvantages of each (Russell 1983). There are several possible study designs that can be used (Box 4.1).

> **Box 4.1 Epidemiological study designs**
>
> *Randomised designs*
>
> - individual patient randomised controlled trials
> - cluster randomised trials
>
> *Non-randomised designs*
>
> - time series designs
> - controlled before-and-after studies
> - before-and-after studies
> - cohort studies
> - case–control studies
> - cross-sectional studies
>
> *Case studies*

The gold standard method for evaluating interventions at the level of the individual is the randomised controlled trial (Cochrane 1979) – the equivalent at the organisational level is the cluster randomised trial. Randomisation is not always possible, usually for practical or ethical reasons (Black 1996). In such circumstances, there are several non-randomised designs that can be considered. We shall focus on the most appropriate and most frequently used designs for studying the way health services are organised and delivered: cluster randomised trials, before-and-after studies, time series analyses, cohort studies and case–control studies.

Definition and theoretical basis

The aim of epidemiological studies is to establish general causal relationships across a population of interest. For example, does the development and dissemination of national clinical guidelines lead to improvements in quality of care in hospitals? The key issue is to identify a research design that enables robust conclusions about whether observed changes are more likely to have been caused by the intervention (for example, dissemination of a national guideline) rather than a simultaneous change in another influential variable (for example, a change in the method of professionals' remuneration). The choice of design will be dependent upon the purpose of the evaluation and the degree of control the researchers have over the delivery of the intervention. In general, researchers should choose a design that minimises potential bias (internal validity) and maximises generalisability (external validity) (Campbell and Stanley 1966; Cook and Campbell 1979). Bias is defined here as any process, at any stage of inference, that tends to produce results or conclusions that differ systematically from the true state of affairs. Generalisability of a study (see Chapter 3) is the degree to which the results hold true for other situations, in particular for routine service delivery (Deeks *et al.* 1995).

While there is a substantial literature about the design, conduct and analysis of evaluations of relatively simple clinical interventions such as drugs, the methods of evaluating complex interventions, such as organisational changes, are less well elucidated. Before discussing the advantages and disadvantages of the various designs, we highlight a number of the likely differences between evaluations of simple and of complex interventions. The evaluation of complex interventions should follow a sequential approach, involving:

- development of a theoretical basis for an intervention being effective
- definition of components of the intervention (using modelling or simulated techniques and qualitative methods)
- exploratory studies to develop further the intervention and plan a definitive evaluative study (using a variety of methods)
- a definitive evaluative study (using quantitative evaluative methods, predominantly randomised designs) (Campbell *et al.* 2000)

This framework demonstrates the interrelationship between quantitative evaluative methods and other methods. It also makes explicit the view that the design and conduct of quantitative evaluative studies should build upon the findings of other research. However, it represents an idealised framework. In some circumstances it is defensible to undertake evaluations without working fully through the earlier stages (for example, when evaluating policy interventions that are being introduced without strong supporting evidence).

Another likely difference between evaluations of simple and complex interventions is that the latter are likely, inherently, to be pragmatic. Schwartz and Lellouch (1967) clarified the distinction between explanatory and pragmatic studies.

Explanatory studies aim to test whether an intervention is efficacious, that is whether the intervention is beneficial under ideal conditions. In explanatory studies, the aim is that contextual factors (e.g. clinical expertise) and other effect modifiers (factors that are known to be related to the size of any effect) are equalised between study groups. Typically they are conducted in highly selected groups of subjects under highly controlled circumstances. Patients withdrawing from such a study may be excluded from analysis. The narrow inclusion criteria and rigid conduct of explanatory studies limit the generalisability of the results to other subjects and contexts.

In contrast, pragmatic studies aim to test whether an intervention is likely to be effective in routine practice by comparing the new procedure with the current regimen; as such they are of more use for developing policy recommendations. Such studies attempt to approximate normal conditions and do not attempt to equalise contextual factors and other effect modifiers in the comparison groups. In pragmatic studies, the contextual and effect-modifying factors therefore become part of the interventions. Such studies are usually conducted on a pre-defined study population, and withdrawals are included within an intention-to-treat analysis. This means that all subjects initially allocated to the intervention group are analysed as intervention subjects irrespective of whether they received the intervention or not. For example, in an evaluation of a new method of organising outpatient clinics, some hospitals may not be able to implement the intervention. In an intention-to-treat analysis, data from all hospitals would be included in the analysis irrespective of whether they could implement the system or not; as a result, the estimates of effect would more likely reflect the effectiveness of the intervention in real-world settings.

Uses of epidemiological studies

Health services are continually evolving. Interventions are frequently introduced to address perceived problems with the way services are organised and delivered. Many of these interventions are based on common sense or political ideology with little supporting research evidence and with the potential for significant opportunity costs if the interventions are ineffective or inefficient (see Chapter 8 for further discussion of opportunity costs). A key role for epidemiology is to evaluate interventions to inform policy decisions prospectively, or to evaluate implemented interventions to ensure that the desired objectives are achieved. Epidemiological methods are useful for estimating the size of the benefits of a new policy or intervention compared to existing practice.

How to undertake epidemiological research

Cluster randomised trials

Randomised trials estimate the impact of an intervention through direct comparison with a randomly allocated control group that either receives no intervention or an alternative intervention. The randomisation process is the best way of ensuring that both known and unknown factors that may independently affect the outcome of an intervention (confounders) are likely to be distributed evenly between the trial groups. As a result, differences observed between groups can be more confidently ascribed to the effects of the intervention rather than to other factors. The same arguments that are used to justify randomised controlled trials of clinical interventions (for example, drugs) are probably at least as salient to the evaluations of organisational interventions. In addition, in our opinion, given the incomplete understanding of potential confounders relating to organisational or professional performance, it is even more difficult to adjust for these in studies of such complex interventions.

While it is possible to conduct randomised trials of organisational interventions which randomise individual patients (see Box 4.2), there is a danger that the treatment given to control individuals will be affected by an organisation's or professional's experience of applying the intervention to other patients in the experimental group; this is known as contamination. If such contamination is likely, the researcher should consider randomising

> ### Box 4.2 Individual patient randomised trials: evaluation of stroke units
>
> In the 1980s there was considerable controversy about the effectiveness of special units to coordinate care for patients with acute strokes. A series of trials randomising around 4,000 patients demonstrated that the provision of organised inpatient care in a 'stroke unit' (characterised by coordinated multidisciplinary rehabilitation, involvement of staff with a special interest in stroke or rehabilitation,

> routine involvement of carers in the rehabilitation process, and
> regular programmes of education and training) led to a 17 per cent
> relative reduction in deaths at one year and a 24 per cent relative
> reduction in death or dependency at one year.
>
> (Stroke Unit Trialists' Collaboration 1999)

organisations or health care professionals rather than individual patients
(see Box 4.3). In such circumstances, data are still often collected about the
process and outcome of care at the individual patient level. Such trials,
which randomise at one level (organisation or professional) and collect data
at a different level (patient), are known as cluster randomised trials (Donner
and Klar 2000; Murray 1998). Cluster randomisation has considerable
implications for the design, power and analysis of studies, which have
frequently been ignored.

Box 4.3 Cluster randomised trial: impact of continuous quality improvement on primary care clinics

Continuous quality improvement (CQI) is a philosophy of continual
improvement of the processes associated with providing a good
service that meets or exceeds customer expectations. Researchers
randomised forty-four US primary care clinics to receive either
support to use CQI methods to improve their preventive care or no
intervention. The study observed that practices which received such
support were more likely to develop system interventions which
followed a CQI process. In addition, professionals in intervention
clinics had higher levels of satisfaction with the way in which preventive services were provided. However, despite a very intensive
intervention there were only marginal improvements of uncertain
clinical significance in actual provision of preventive services.

(Solberg *et al.* 1998; Kottke *et al.* 2000; Solberg *et al.* 2000)

Design considerations

The main design considerations concern the level of randomisation and
whether to include baseline measurement. Frequently researchers need to
trade off the likelihood of contamination at lower levels of randomisation
against decreasing numbers of clusters and increasing logistical problems at

higher levels of randomisation. For example, in a study of an educational intervention in secondary care settings, potential levels of randomisation include the individual clinician, the ward, the clinical service or directorate, and the hospital. Randomisation at the level of the hospital would minimise the risk of contamination but dramatically increase the number of hospitals required. Randomisation at the level of the individual clinician would decrease the number of hospitals required, but there would be considerable risk of contamination of clinicians working in the same wards or speciality areas. Under such circumstances, researchers may choose to randomise at the level of hospital wards or groups of wards (if there is a risk of contamination because of shared policies and cross-ward cover of staff across same-speciality wards within the same hospital).

Commonly, in cluster randomised trials, relatively few clusters (e.g. hospitals) are available for randomisation. Under these circumstances, there is an increased danger of imbalance in performance between study and control groups due to chance. Baseline measurements can be used to assess the adequacy of the allocation process. Baseline measures of performance are useful because they also provide an estimate of the magnitude of a problem. Low-performance scores prior to the intervention indicate that there is much room for improvement, whereas high-performance scores indicate that there is little room for improvement (known as a ceiling effect). In addition, baseline measures could be used as a stratifying or matching variable, or be incorporated into the analysis to increase statistical power (see below). These potential benefits have to be weighed against the increased costs and duration of studies incorporating baseline measurements and concerns about testing effects (introduction of potential bias due to sensitisation of the study subjects during baseline measurement) (Campbell and Stanley 1966).

Sample size calculations

A fundamental assumption of the standard statistics used to analyse individual patient randomised trials is that the outcome for an individual patient is completely unrelated to that for any other patient – they are said to be 'independent'. This assumption is violated, however, when cluster randomisation is adopted, because two patients within any one cluster are more likely to respond in a similar manner than two patients in different clusters. For example, the management of patients in a single hospital is more likely to be consistent than management of patients between hospitals. The main disadvantage of adopting a cluster randomised design is that it is not as statistically efficient and has lower statistical power than an individual patient randomised trial of the same size.

Sample sizes for cluster randomised trials therefore need to be inflated to adjust for clustering. A statistical measure of the extent of clustering is known as the 'intracluster correlation coefficient' (ICC) which is based on the relationship of the between-cluster to within-cluster variance (Donner and Koval 1980). Both the ICC and the cluster size influence the inflation required, which can be considerable, especially if the average cluster size is large. The extra numbers of patients required can be achieved by increasing either the number of clusters in the study or the number of patients per cluster. Increasing the number of clusters is the more efficient method (Diwan *et al.* 1992). In general, little additional power is gained from increasing the number of patients per cluster above fifty. Researchers often have to trade off the logistic difficulties and costs associated with recruitment of extra clusters against those associated with increasing the number of patients per cluster.

Researchers rarely have direct estimates of the ICC from the study population of interest when planning studies. Under these circumstances they can either undertake pilot work to calculate an ICC, or they can seek estimates derived from previous studies of similar populations. Unfortunately, there are relatively few published estimates (Ukoumunne *et al.* 1999; Campbell *et al.* 2000a) and researchers need to consider the likely generalisability of the ICCs to their population of interest.

Analysis

There are three approaches to the analysis of cluster randomised trials: analysis at cluster level, the adjustment of standard tests, and advanced statistical techniques using data recorded at both the individual and cluster level (Donner 1998; Murray 1998). No consensus exists as to which approach should be used. The most appropriate option will depend on a number of factors, including the research question; the unit of inference; the study design; whether the researchers wish to adjust for other relevant variables (co-variables) at the individual or cluster level; the type and distribution of outcome measures; the number of clusters randomised; the size of cluster and variability of cluster size; and statistical resources available in the research team. Worked examples comparing these different analytical strategies have been reported (Campbell *et al.* 2000b; Mollison *et al.* 2000).

Before-and-after studies

Before-and-after studies measure performance before and after the introduction of an intervention. Observed differences in performance, not otherwise explained, are assumed to be due to the intervention (Figure 4.1).

These studies are relatively simple to conduct but are methodologically weak because secular trends or other concurrent changes make it difficult to attribute observed changes to the intervention being studied. In general, uncontrolled before-and-after studies should not be used to evaluate the

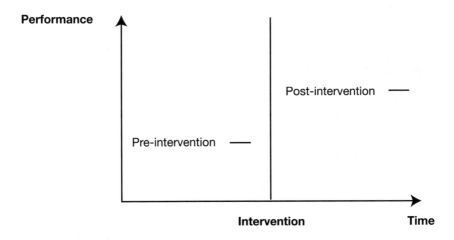

Figure 4.1 Uncontrolled-before-and-after study

effects of SDO interventions, and the results of studies using such designs have to be interpreted with great caution.

A modification is to introduce a comparison group or setting to act as a control. In controlled before-and-after studies, the researcher attempts to identify a control population that has similar characteristics and performance to the study population, and collects data in both populations before and after the intervention is applied to the study population (Figure 4.2).

Analysis compares post-intervention performance or change scores in the study and control groups, and observed differences are assumed to be due to

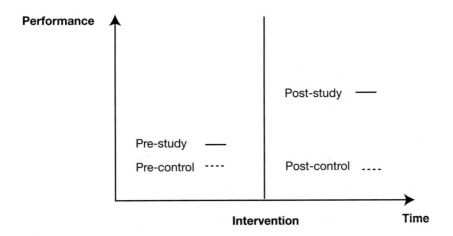

Figure 4.2 Controlled-before-and-after study

the intervention (Box 4.4). The importance of incorporating a control group was demonstrated by Lipsey and Wilson (1993), who reviewed forty-five

> ### Box 4.4 Controlled before-and-after study: evaluation of a hospital picture archiving and communication system
>
> The aim was to establish the impact of introducing a hospital-wide picture archiving and communication system (PACS) that comprised digital acquisition, storage, and transmission of radiological images via a hospital-wide network to 150 workstations. A controlled before-and-after design was the most robust research design that could be employed given that a randomised trial would have required allocation at the hospital level and the PACS was being introduced in only one hospital. Data were also collected at five other control hospitals, selected by similarity of size and activity.
>
> The introduction of PACS was associated with several significant gains, for example, an improvement in image availability (97.7 per cent versus 86.9 per cent) and thus reduction in repeat image ordering which was not observed in the five control hospitals. However, this change was not reflected for patients in the hospital where the new system was introduced, who did not spend less time waiting for their radiology results compared to patients in the control hospitals.
>
> (Bryan *et al.* 1999)

meta-analyses of psychological, educational and behavioural interventions and noted that the observed effects from uncontrolled before-and-after studies were greater than those from controlled studies.

While controlled before-and-after studies should protect against secular trends and concurrent interventions, it is often difficult to identify a comparable control group. Even in apparently well matched control and study groups, performances at baseline often differ. Under these circumstances, 'within group' analyses are often undertaken (where change from baseline is compared within both groups separately and where the assumption is made that if the change in the intervention group is significant and the change in the control group is not, the intervention has had an effect). Such analyses are inappropriate for a number of reasons. First, the baseline imbalance suggests that the control group is not truly comparable and may not experience the same secular trends or concurrent interventions as the intervention group; thus any apparent effect of the intervention may be spurious. Second, there is no direct comparison between study and control groups (Campbell and Stanley 1966). Another common analytical problem in practice is that researchers fail to recognise clustering of data when interventions are delivered at an organisational level and data are collected at the individual patient level.

Time series analyses

Time series designs attempt to detect whether an intervention has had an effect significantly greater than the underlying secular trend (Cook and Campbell 1979). They are useful for evaluating the effects of interventions when it is difficult to randomise, such as the impact of the dissemination of national guidelines or mass media campaigns (Box 4.5). Data are collected

---

Box 4.5 Time series design: evaluation of impact of national clinical guidelines

A time series design was used to evaluate the effectiveness of guidelines for Caesarean section in Ontario. Monthly data from hospitals from April 1982 to March 1986 provided pre-intervention information about antenatal practice. The guidelines were disseminated to all obstetricians in March–June 1986, and the effect was assessed by analysing monthly data from April 1986 to March 1988.

After release of the guidelines, there was no clear, dramatic decrease in the rates of Caesarean section. However, statistical analysis revealed that prior to the guidelines the monthly increase had been 0.029 per cent, whereas afterwards there was a monthly decrease of 0.04 per cent, a potential effect from the guidelines of 0.13 fewer Caesarean sections per 100 deliveries each year.

(Lomas et al. 1989)

---

at several times before and after the intervention; the data collected before the intervention allow the underlying trend and cyclical (seasonal) effects to be estimated. The data collected after the intervention allow the intervention effect to be estimated while taking account of the underlying secular trends (Figure 4.3).

To strengthen the design, a comparison group or setting can be incorporated, referred to as multiple time series design. For example, the impact of a regional mass media campaign to change people's behaviour can be compared with the changes taking place for other reasons in another region in which no mass media campaign was carried out.

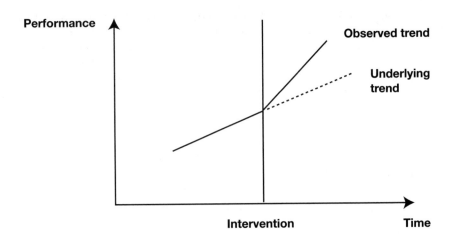

Figure 4.3 Time series analysis

There are several statistical techniques that can be used for analysis depending on the characteristics of the data, the number of data points available and whether autocorrelation is present (Cook and Campbell 1979). Autocorrelation refers to the situation whereby data points collected close in time are likely to be more similar to each other than to data points collected far apart. For example, for any given month, the waiting times in hospitals are likely to be more similar to waiting times in adjacent months than to waiting times twelve months previously. It is necessary to collect enough data points prior to the intervention to be convinced that a stable estimate of the underlying secular trend has been obtained. When designing a time series analysis, there is often a trade-off between the number and stability of data points. The time interval between successive data points should be chosen with care. The interval should be short enough to pick up secular trends but not so short that any intervention effect disappears in the background 'noise'. For example, if the intervention is believed to affect only the first four or five months after its introduction, then it would be appropriate to use 'months' as the data points. Using weekly data in this situation may show large variability between data points and hence make it difficult to identify an intervention effect.

Cohort studies

When randomisation is not possible, another possible design that can be used is a cohort study. A cohort study follows a group of people who have all shared a common experience or exposure, such as undergoing a particular treatment, and compares their outcome with a similar group who have received some other form of care (or no formal care). The analysis compares the incidence of the outcome of interest in the two cohorts, in order to determine whether an association exists between the intervention and the outcome. In essence, they are non-randomised trials in that there is no attempt by the researcher to allocate individuals to a particular intervention on a random basis. Instead they make use of the naturally occurring differences or variations in the way services are organised and interventions are used (Box 4.6).

Box 4.6 Cohort study: the effectiveness of a helicopter emergency medical service

Helicopter ambulance services have been introduced widely over the past three decades in the USA, and more recently in Germany and Norway. The introduction of a similar method of delivering emergency care in London provided an opportunity to assess its impact on the outcome of patients. Two cohorts were recruited: those patients attended by the helicopter emergency service during a two-year period and those cared for by the existing land ambulance paramedics – over the same period. All survivors were followed up two and six months after their injury by means of mailed questionnaires.

Comparison of outcomes was adjusted for possible confounding factors: age, sex, injury severity score, Glasgow Coma Score, Revised Trauma Score, Abbreviated Injury Scale, body region score and type of incident. There was no evidence of reduced disability or better functional status in those attended by the helicopter service despite the extra cost incurred.

(Brazier et al. 1996)

For example, hospitals may differ as to which staff take blood from patients – in some it is the junior doctors and in others a specialised member of staff known as a phlebotomist. The relative merits of these two arrangements could be explored by comparing the proportion of adequate samples obtained in hospitals using doctors and in hospitals using phlebotomists.

Clearly, in the absence of randomisation, it is possible that any observed differences might have nothing to do with the intervention being studied but may arise because of other differences (so-called confounding factors). In non-randomised comparisons it is necessary, therefore, to consider the influence of potential confounders. Those factors that are known to be influential can, in theory, be measured, and any difference between the study and control groups can be taken into account in the statistical analysis. Inevitably, there may be confounders that are unrecognised and cannot therefore be measured and adjusted for. The consequence is that the results of a cohort study (or non-randomised trial) must be interpreted with care as they may be subject to bias (poor internal validity).

Cohort studies can be conducted in two ways, prospectively or retrospectively. The difference is in the timing of the cohort of patients' experience of the intervention being evaluated. In a prospective design, patients are recruited to the study in the present and then followed into the future to determine the impact of the intervention. In a retrospective design, a cohort of patients who experienced the intervention at some time in the past are identified and their outcome is assessed in the present day. The advantage of the latter is that information on the long-term effect of the intervention (maybe ten or twenty years) can be assessed without having to wait a long time. The disadvantages are that detailed information of an intervention received may be lacking (unless there are good historical records) and the researcher has no control of what information on the individuals was collected in the past, or how it was collected. Dependence on patients' or clinicians' recollection may introduce serious biases.

Case–control studies

Case–control studies take as their starting point the outcome of interest, such as an adverse event resulting from health care. Subjects suffering such an event are designated 'cases' and those without are designated 'controls'. Data are then assembled on the prior exposure or experiences of all subjects. The analysis compares the probability of prior exposure of cases to that of controls (Box 4.7). For example, hospital ward managers may want to investigate the

---

Box 4.7 Case–control study: effectiveness of a syringe exchange programme

A case–control design was used to assess the effectiveness of a syringe exchange programme in reducing the incidence of blood-borne viruses in injecting drug users. The programme had been implemented in the community three years before the evaluation. Within a study population of intravenous drug users, the prior use of the exchange was compared in cases with confirmed hepatitis B or C and appropriately matched controls without infection. The researchers demonstrated that non-use of the

> exchange was associated with a sixfold higher risk of hepatitis B and a sevenfold higher risk of hepatitis C, once potential confounding factors had been adjusted for.
>
> (Hagan *et al.* 1995)

reasons for elderly patients falling and injuring themselves. Cases would be defined as those experiencing such injuries, while controls would be selected from other patients. Usually controls are selected to be similar to cases in some regards such as age and sex. However, any factors which are used for 'matching' of controls to cases cannot be investigated as possible factors associated with the outcome. For example, if cases and controls were matched for age, it would not be possible to see if falls were associated with the age of the patient.

Case–control studies only reveal whether or not there is an association – they cannot determine whether such an association is causal or not. However, they are relatively quick and cheap to perform, so provide a useful initial mode of enquiry. Given that case–control studies work backwards from the outcome of care (unlike cohort studies which start from the inception of care), they are limited in their use to investigating the reasons for an adverse event or poor performance.

Limitations of epidemiological methods

Randomised trials should only be considered when there is genuine uncertainty about the effectiveness of an intervention. While we argue that randomised trials are the optimal design for evaluating interventions to improve the organisation of health services, they have a number of drawbacks. They can be logistically difficult, especially if the researchers are using complex designs to evaluate more than one intervention, or if cluster randomisation requires the recruitment of large numbers of clusters. They are undoubtedly methodologically challenging and require a multidisciplinary approach to plan and conduct adequately. They are also time-consuming, expensive and can rarely be completed in less than two years.

Critics of randomised trials frequently express concerns that the tight inclusion criteria of trials, or the artificial constraints placed upon participants, limit the generalisability of the findings. While this is a particular concern in efficacy (explanatory) studies of health technologies, it is likely to be less of a problem when studying organisational interventions which, by their nature, will tend to be pragmatic.

The main limitation of non-randomised designs is that the lack of randomised controls threatens internal validity and increases the likelihood of plausible rival hypotheses. Cook and Campbell (1979) suggest that:

> Estimating the internal validity of a relationship is a deductive process in which the investigator has to systematically think through how each of the internal validity threats may have influenced the data. Then the investigator has to examine the data to test which relevant threats can be ruled out. ... When all of the threats can plausibly be eliminated it is possible to make confident conclusions about whether a relationship is probably causal.

In non-randomised designs, there are potentially greater threats to internal validity and less ability to account for them. The design and conduct of non-randomised studies are at least as methodologically challenging as the design and conduct of randomised trials. As with randomised trials, the external validity of non-randomised studies may also be poor if they are conducted in a small number of study sites not representative of the population to which the researcher wishes to generalise.

Cohort and case–control studies can provide valuable insights into the impact of organisational factors that are associated with an outcome. The results from such studies are useful for generating hypotheses for further study, and for determining the extent of success of the implementation of an intervention in the wider population of subjects of interest. However, making causal inferences can be difficult because the populations to be compared may differ in characteristics that affect the outcomes being measured – characteristics other than the interventions to be compared. If the evaluator cannot identify or measure these differences, nothing can be done to ameliorate the resulting bias.

Further reading

General

Boruch, R. F. and Foley, E. (2000) 'The honestly experimental society: sites and other entities as units of allocation and analysis in randomized trials', in L. Bickman (ed.) *Validity and Social Experimentation*, Thousand Oaks CA: Sage.

Cochrane, A. L. (1979) *Effectiveness and Efficiency: Random Reflections on Health Services*, London: Nuffield Provincial Hospitals Trust.

Oakley, A. (1998) 'Experimentation and social interventions: a forgotten but important history', *British Medical Journal*, 317: 1239–42.

UK Medical Research Council (2000) *A Framework for Development and Evaluation of RCTs for Complex Interventions to Improve Health*, London: Medical Research Council (available from http://www.mrc.ac.uk/mrc_cpr.pdf).

Individual patient randomised trials

Boruch, R. F. (1997) *Randomized Experiments for Planning and Evaluation: A Practical Guide*, Thousand Oaks CA: Sage.

Pocock, S. J. (1983) *Clinical Trials: a Practical Approach*, New York: Wiley.

Cluster randomised trials

Donner, A. and Klar, N. (2000) *Design and Analysis of Cluster Randomisation Trials in Health Research*, London: Arnold.

Murray, D. M. (1998) *The Design and Analysis of Group Randomised Trials*, Oxford: Oxford University Press.

Ukoumunne, O. C., Gulliford, M. C., Chinn, S., Sterne, J. A. C. and Burney, P. G. J. (1999) 'Methods for evaluating area-wide and organization based interventions in health and health care: a systematic review', *Health Technology Assessment*, 3, 5.

A public domain cluster randomised sample size calculator is available from: http://www.abdn.ac.uk/hsru/epp/ss.hti

Non-randomised designs

Cook, T. D. and Campbell, D. T. (1979) *Quasi-experimentation: Design and Analysis Issues for Field Settings*, Chicago: Rand McNally.

Campbell, D. T. and Stanley, J. C. (1966) *Experimental and Quasi-experimental Designs for Research*, Chicago: Rand McNally.

Rothman, K. J. and Greenland, S. (1998) *Modern Epidemiology*, 2nd edn, Philadelphia: Lippincott Williams and Wilkins.

References

Black, N. A. (1996) 'Why we need observational studies to evaluate the effectiveness of health care', *British Medical Journal*, 312: 1215–18.

Brazier, J., Nicholls, J. and Snooks, H. (1996) 'The cost and effectiveness of the London helicopter emergency medical service', *Journal of Health Services Research and Policy*, 1: 232–7.

Bryan, S., Weatherburn, G., Buxton, M., Watkins, J., Keen, J. and Muris, N. (1999) 'Evaluation of a hospital produce activity and communication system', *Journal of Health Services Research and Policy*, 4: 204–9.

Campbell, D. T. and Stanley, J. C. (1966) *Experimental and Quasi-experimental Designs for Research*, Chicago: Rand McNally.

Campbell, M., Fitzpatrick, R., Haines, A., Kinmonth, A. L., Sandercock, P., Spiegelhalter, D. and Tyrer, P. (2000) 'Framework for design and evaluation of complex interventions to improve health', *British Medical Journal*, 321: 694–6.

Campbell, M. K., Grimshaw, J. M. and Steen, I. N. (2000a) 'Sample size calculations for cluster randomised trials', *Journal of Health Services Research and Policy*, 5: 12–16.

Campbell, M. K., Mollison, J., Steen, N., Grimshaw, J. M. and Eccles, M. P. (2000b) 'Analysis of cluster randomised trials in primary care: a practical approach', *Family Practice*, 17: 192–6.

Cochrane, A. L. (1979) *Effectiveness and Efficiency: Random Reflections on Health Services*, London: Nuffield Provincial Hospitals Trust.

Cook, T. D. and Campbell, D. T. (1979) *Quasi-experimentation: Design and Analysis Issues for Field Settings*, Chicago: Rand McNally.

Deeks, J. J., Glanvill, J. M. and Sheldon, T. A. (1995) *Undertaking Systematic Reviews of Research on Effectiveness*, York: NHS Centre for Reviews and Dissemination.

Diwan, V. K., Eriksson, B., Sterky, G. and Tomson, G. (1992) 'Randomisation by group in studying the effect of drug information in primary care', *International Journal of Epidemiology*, 21: 124–30.

Donner, A. (1998) 'Some aspects of the design and analysis of cluster randomisation trials', *Applied Statistics*, 47: 95–113.

Donner, A. and Klar, N. (2000) *Design and Analysis of Cluster Randomisation Trials in Health Research*, London: Arnold.

Donner, A. and Koval, J. J. (1980) 'The estimation of intraclass correlation in the analysis of family data', *Biometrics*, 36: 19–25.

Hagan, H., Des Jarlais, D. C., Friedman, S. R., Purchase, D. and Alter, M. J. (1995) 'Reduced risk of hepatitis B and hepatitis C among injection drug users in the Tacoma Syringe Exchange Program', *American Journal of Public Health*, 85: 1531–7.

Kottke, T. E., Solberg, L. I., Brekke, M. L., Magnan, S. and Amundson, G. M. (2000) 'Clinician satisfaction with a preventive services implementation trial: the IMPROVE project', *American Journal of Preventive Medicine*, 18: 219–24.

Lipsey, M. W. and Wilson, D. B. (1993) 'The efficacy of psychological, educational and behavioural treatment: confirmation from meta-analysis', *American Psychologist*, 48: 1181–209.

Lomas, J., Anderson, G. M., Dominick-Pierre, K., Vayda, E., Enkin, M. W. and Hannah, W. J. (1989) 'Do practice guidelines guide practice? The effect of a consensus statement on the practice of physicians', *New England Journal of Medicine*, 321: 1306–11.

Mollison, J., Simpson, J. A., Campbell, M. K. and Grimshaw, J. M. (2000) 'Comparison of analytical methods for cluster randomised trials: an example from a primary care setting', *Journal of Epidemiology and Biostatistics*, 5: 339–46.

Murray, D. M. (1998) *The Design and Analysis of Group Randomised Trials*, Oxford: Oxford University Press.

Russell, I. T. (1983) 'The evaluation of a computerised tomography: a review of research methods', in A. J. Culyer and B. Horisberger (eds) *Economic and Medical Evaluation of Health Care Technologies*, Berlin: Springer-Verlag.

Schwartz, D. and Lellouch, J. (1967) 'Explanatory and pragmatic attitudes in clinical trials', *Journal of Chronic Diseases*, 20, 637–48.

Solberg, L. I., Kottke, T. E. and Brekke, M. L. (1998) 'Will primary care clinics organize themselves to improve the delivery of preventive services? A randomized controlled trial', *Preventive Medicine*, 27: 623–31.

Solberg, L. I., Kottke, T. E., Brekke, M. L., Magnan, S., Davidson, G., Calomeni, C. A., Conn, S. A., Amundson, G. M. and Nelson, A. F. (2000) 'Failure of a continuous quality improvement intervention to increase the delivery of preventive services: a randomized trial', *Effective Clinical Practice*, 3: 105–15.

Stroke Unit Trialists' Collaboration (1999) 'Organised inpatient (stroke unit) care for stroke (Cochrane Review)', in *The Cochrane Library*, issue 4, Oxford: Update Software.

Ukoumunne, O. C., Gulliford, M. C., Chinn, S., Sterne, J. A. C. and Burney, P. G. J. (1999) 'Methods for evaluating area-wide and organisation based interventions in health and health care: a systematic review', *Health Technology Assessment*, 3: 5.

Chapter 5

Organisational psychology

John Arnold

Introduction

Psychology as a discipline concerns the description, explanation and prediction of behaviour, thoughts and emotions. Organisational psychologists draw upon a range of theoretical and methodological traditions in seeking to address issues to do with human behaviour, thoughts and emotions at work. Most of this work is not specific to health care settings, but is designed to be generalisable to many contexts. Existing research and theory have something to say of practical importance in health service delivery and organisation, even though it is rarely framed in ways that exactly match health service managers' day-to-day concerns or vocabulary. The methods used by organisational psychologists permit the investigation of a wide range of topics and a choice of underlying research philosophy. There are many published examples of organisational psychology making significant potential and actual contributions to health service delivery and organisation, particularly concerning aspects of human resource management.

Definition and theoretical basis

There are a number of sub-disciplines within psychology, including elements drawn from the arts, humanities, and the biological and physical sciences as well as social science. One way of viewing the sub-disciplines is as follows.

- Biological psychology examines the relationships between brain and body and the neurological and physiological ways in which psychological processes are manifested.
- Social psychology considers the ways in which the behaviour, thoughts and emotions of individuals and groups influence, and are influenced by, their social contexts.
- Personality psychology focuses on the nature, configuration and expression of the general psychological characteristics of humanity and the specific psychological characteristics of individuals.

- Cognitive psychology involves the study of thought processes such as problem solving and memory, as well as issues on the border with biological psychology such as the processing of visual and auditory information.
- Developmental psychology concerns how individuals unfold in all the above areas, mainly during childhood but also during the adult years.

Within psychology there are a number of areas of application which draw upon concepts, theories and techniques from the five sub-disciplines described above. These areas of application also boast some theories, concepts and techniques of their own, which to a limited extent feed back into psychology more generally. One of these areas of application is termed 'organisational psychology'. And normally this organisational context is that of work. In fact, the usual name in mainland Europe for this area is 'work and organisational psychology'. In North America it is 'industrial/organisational (I/O) psychology'. In the United Kingdom alone, it is often also referred to as occupational psychology. There are other names as well, each with subtle messages about what is included and excluded. The term 'organisational psychology' tends to exclude elements close to physical science such as ergonomics. But even that is not a hard and fast rule.

The dominant paradigm in psychology is borrowed from the physical sciences. It tends to spill over to a greater or lesser extent in the applied areas, including organisational psychology. It has consequences for the ways in which problems and issues are framed, the methods used to investigate them, the way that research is reported and the kinds of conclusions that are drawn. For the sake of brevity it will be referred to here as the positivist paradigm (see Chapter 1). It emphasises the objective definition of problems, precise quantitative measurement, and cause/effect models of human behaviour (James and James 1989).

But there are alternative paradigms. These can be referred to under the general name of interpretive. The interpretive paradigm is not dominant in organisational psychology, but it does have more than a foothold. It emphasises the subjective nature of knowledge and the importance of the accounts people create of their actions. It usually involves qualitative rather than quantitative data. Table 5.1 compares the two paradigms.

The tension between the two general paradigms is evident in other disciplines as well as psychology – for example, sociology (see Chapters 2 and 3). The two paradigms coexist rather uneasily in organisational psychology, though there have been attempts to bring them together (Taber 1991).

The notions of validity and reliability are central to much of organisational psychology research (Anastasi 1988), reflecting the dominance of the positivist paradigm. Validity refers to the extent to which a research method or data collection tool measures what it is supposed to measure. Sometimes

Table 5.1 The positivist and interpretive paradigms in organisational psychology

The positivist paradigm	The interpretive paradigm
Objective, detached researcher	*Subjective, involved researcher*
Assumes that, with care, what is being researched can be objectively assessed without the research process having any impact on what is being researched.	Assumes that knowledge is subjectively defined and that the research task is to get involved with people to hear their subjective accounts.
Hypothesis-testing	*Hypothesis-generating*
Derives testable hypotheses, usually from theory and usually concerning causes and effects, and seeks to ascertain the extent to which they are supported or falsified by the research data.	Seeks to describe and analyse possible themes and nuances of meaning that can be interpreted from research data.
Nomothetic	*Idiographic*
Seeks general rules of behaviour, thoughts or emotions, applicable to all members of large populations within specified situational parameters.	Seeks to describe and analyse how an individual behaves, thinks or feels in his or her unique way.
Parsimonious	*Richness, complexity*
Seeks to describe, explain or predict using the simplest configuration and smallest number of variables necessary.	Seeks to generate possibilities, ideas, perhaps using a large number of constructs which interrelate in complex and perhaps unpredictable ways.
Experimental, decontextualised	*Non-experimental, contextualised*
Attempts to investigate issues under controlled conditions so that the causes and effects of certain factors can be evaluated.	Attempts to analyse people and events in their naturally occurring context, without seeking to manipulate the conditions to which they are exposed.
Quantitative measurement, statistics	*Qualitative data, interpretation*
Data are usually quantitative, and assumed to measure something that objectively exists. Data are analysed to test hypotheses using sometimes complex statistical techniques.	Data are usually qualitative, and assumed to be reflecting narratives, accounts given by specific people in specific circumstances. Analysis is through suggesting interpretations of textual or verbal data.

validity is assessed with reference to the theory upon which the measurement is based – so-called construct or content validity. On other occasions it is gauged against an outcome measure of practical importance. This latter form is referred to as criterion validity and is common, for example, in the evaluation of psychometric tests. The validity of tests of personality characteristics or mental ability is often assessed in terms of whether they predict job performance, rather than whether they accurately reflect the components of the theoretical constructs upon which they are based. This kind of pragmatic approach is quite prevalent in organisational psychology. It reflects the fact that many organisational psychologists operate in a commercial environment where they sell their services to clients who are usually aiming to improve performance and/or profitability. It also means that validity can be quite context-specific (for example, confined to certain kinds of job) rather than being an inherent property of the method.

Reliability refers to the extent to which a method or data-collection tool produces consistent results. This may be expressed as a correlation, reflecting the extent to which the scores of a group of people remain constant relative to each other over a short period of time (usually a matter of a few weeks), or on the level of agreement, reflecting the extent to which scores remain the same. Where the measurement tool consists of a number of items all tapping the same construct (for example, a set of questions assessing a person's commitment to their employing organisation), reliability may also be expressed in terms of an alpha coefficient which reflects the extent to which responses to those questions 'hang together' in a way which suggests that a single underlying construct is being assessed.

Validity is of course construed somewhat differently by adherents of the interpretive paradigm. Because this approach emphasises the subjective and context-specific nature of knowledge, validity is seen much more as the extent to which a researcher's interpretation of data is plausible and/or useful to various audiences who might have a stake in it. This form of validity is much more difficult to ascertain than the positivist one, and reports of interpretive research rarely include statistics supporting the integrity of the research measures, in the way that positivist reports more routinely do.

Uses

There are two ways of looking at the uses of organisational psychology. The first is to look at the usual topic areas included within organisational psychology. Table 5.2 derives from an analysis of papers published in the leading British academic journal in organisational psychology. It has an international reputation and readership. Other journals in the field would show a slightly different range and frequency of topics, but the list can nevertheless be considered a useful guide to what organisational psychology is about.

In a sense, one of the most telling elements is that 16 per cent of articles fell in the 'Other' category. This indicates the great range of subjects included in organisational psychology, for example, organisational change, training, management development and decision making. One could infer from the table that much of the focus of organisational psychology is on individuals as opposed to organisations. This is broadly true, but perhaps not quite as much so as it might seem. Certainly the focus is often on individuals, but sometimes data on individuals' behaviour, thoughts and emotions are investigated in conjunction with measures at an organisational

Table 5.2 Topic areas of papers published in *Journal of Occupational and Organisational Psychology*, 1995–9

Topic area	Percentage of published papers	Trend over period 1995–9
Stress/burnout	18	Down
Selection and assessment	15	Down
Personality/individual differences	9	
Commitment/motivation	8	Down
Unemployment	5	
Career development	5	Up
Culture/climate	5	Up
Gender issues	5	
Job demands/performance	4	
Leadership	4	Up
Teams/groups	3	
Emotion/mood	3	
Others	16	

Source: Sparrow, personal communication, 2000

level, such as the performance of the organisation. Also, aspects of the micro- and macro-environments that organisations create for their members are often included in organisational psychology research. Nevertheless, most of organisational psychology does treat individuals or groups as the key concern, rather than the organisation. This might be quite in tune with the times since, thanks to teleworking and outsourcing, more and more work is becoming relatively independent of organisational contexts (Arthur and Rousseau 1996).

The second way of looking at the uses of organisational psychology is to consider the kind of issues that can be addressed. Ten such questions are:

1   *What is the nature of the phenomenon in question?* For example: how many different types of organisational commitment can be identified? What are the fundamental dimensions of personality at work? Are culture and climate the same thing?

2   *Development and validation of measures or techniques.* For example: a questionnaire-based measure on which people report the extent to which they exhibit the symptoms of burnout; the development of a method of scoring life history data as a tool in employee selection; the development of a questionnaire to assess the 'climate for innovation' in an organisation.

3   *What factors influence the phenomenon in question?* For example: what are the roles of interpersonal conflict and highly responsible work in

determining levels of stress? What is it about being unemployed that tends to lead to anxiety and depression? Which aspects of interpersonal dynamics in teams most strongly influence the team's success?

4   *Proposal and/or demonstration of a new theory or theoretical ideas.* For example: the links between job satisfaction, organisational commitment and intention to leave the organisation; construing employee selection as a social process rather than a technical task.

5   *Tests of one or more theories.* For example: do theories of leadership based on individual charisma apply in collectivist cultures? Does a theory of career success based upon organisational opportunities predict career success better than a theory based upon individuals' attributes?

6   *What is the impact of an intervention?* For example: does the introduction of a new assessment centre lead to the selection of higher-performing employees, and if so how? In what respects, if any, does training in diversity affect people's attitudes to minority groups at work? What is the impact of stress management training on how much stress people experience, and how they deal with it?

7   *What are the consequences of particular psychological states or characteristics?* For example: Does feeling committed to an organisation lead people to work harder, and/or put themselves out more? How does the experience of stress affect a person's overall work performance and mental health? Are some personality characteristics more suited than others to top-level management work?

8   *How do groups of people differ from each other?* For example: do female leaders tend to behave differently from male leaders? Are nurses more stressed than doctors? Do people from different cultures expect different behaviour in job interviews?

9   *How do people make sense of their work and their workplace?* For example: how do people account for their reasons for moving from employment to self-employment? How do senior managers use constructs associated with gender to account for the behaviour of colleagues?

10   *How replicable/generalisable is a particular finding?* For example: are job interviews necessarily a poor way of selecting people? Do the negative effects of performance-related pay apply to middle managers as well as first-level supervisors? Is the psychological impact of unemployment the same in an area with a lot of unemployment as in an area with little?

All of these types of issues can be found in articles published in organisational psychology journals. However, tests of theory and of the causes and consequences of psychological phenomena tend to be the most prevalent.

How to undertake organisational psychology research

One consequence of the relatively decontextualised nature of much organisational psychology is that little of it has been *both* conducted in health service settings *and* designed primarily to address health service issues. However, quite a lot that has taken place in health service settings has implications for service delivery and organisation, even though it was designed to investigate issues of broader application or theoretical nature. Boxes 5.1–5.5 demonstrate the kinds of issues psychologists tend to investigate and the ways in which they do so.

Some organisational psychology research is laboratory-based and experimental. That is, a particular phenomenon is investigated using comparisons between groups of people subjected to different treatments under controlled conditions. Assignment of participants to experimental groups is often random, though the participants as a group are rarely a random sample of the relevant wider population. Other research is field-based and experimental. Experimental studies are notable by their absence, reflecting the difficulties in finding or creating situations that lend themselves to experimental investigation in field settings. Sometimes organisations allow psychologists to set up an experiment in the workplace, in order to compare the impact of different interventions. More often, field experiments are naturally occurring: that is to say, they capitalise upon developments that are happening anyway (see Chapter 4). For example, a hospital might change its pattern of shiftwork in some wards but not others. Assignment of people to experimental conditions is unlikely to be random in field experiments, and sometimes it is difficult to gain access early enough to obtain pre-intervention measures.

Surveys involve the collection and analysis of data without any attempt to intervene in naturally occurring conditions. For example, Hemingway and Smith (1999) used a quantitative survey to investigate whether aspects of organisational climate and individuals' levels of stress predicted absence, turnover and injury amongst nurses. Systematic comparison of the effects upon people of different interventions is difficult to achieve in surveys, though the inclusion of a range of carefully chosen questions can go some way towards it, especially if the survey is longitudinal – that is, data are collected at more than one point in time (see Box 5.1). So, for example, obtaining data about the pattern of shiftwork a respondent experiences and how long they have experienced it may help to identify possible effects on the person.

Organisational psychologists also use research designs associated with the interpretive paradigm. For example, some engage in action research, where data are collected in a participative style and fed back to the providers with the aim of acting upon the findings and evaluating the outcomes of any such actions (see Chapter 11). Qualitative research is

> **Box 5.1 Assessment of occupational stress in doctors**
>
> An example of a survey-based, complex set of quantitative compar-
> isons between groups and between variables is provided by Swanson
> and colleagues (1998). They obtained questionnaire data from 986
> hospital doctors and general practitioners in Scotland in an attempt
> to examine the extent of occupational stress (especially concerning
> the work/family interface) and the extent to which it varied with
> gender and domestic responsibilities (labelled 'role complexity' by
> the authors).
>
> Among other findings, the authors report that men reported
> working longer hours than women, and hospital doctors more than
> GPs. The amount of domestic work undertaken was much greater for
> those with families and for women, irrespective of whether they had
> a family. There was also an interaction between gender and role
> complexity, such that with increasing family responsibilities the
> amount of domestic work undertaken by women increased much
> more than the amount undertaken by men. Nevertheless, the amount
> of stress experienced concerning the work/family interface was
> scarcely greater for women than for men, and women scored at least
> as high as men on job satisfaction.
>
> (Swanson et al. 1998)

marked by attempts to explore in depth the experiences of individuals and
the meanings they attach to them and possible interpretations of them (see
Chapter 3). Like a survey, there is no attempt systematically to manipulate
the conditions people experience but, unlike a survey, the emphasis is not
upon collecting information that approximates to an objective reality, nor is
it on establishing causality. The role of the researcher is to elicit and perhaps
provoke ideas, accounts and explanations.

It can be said that much of organisational psychology aspires to be experimental. Although that aspiration is by no means always achieved, it reflects
the natural science roots of psychology. Schaubroeck and Kuehn (1992) for
example, reviewed the research design used in 199 studies published in three
leading North American journals during 1989 and 1990. They concluded
that:

> a majority of published studies were conducted in the field, although
> labwork comprises near one-third of the research. Half of the published
> research was experimental, and most studies endeavoured to support a
> specific refutable hypothesis. ... Most studies minimised common

method factors by using diverse data sources. On the downside, a majority of field studies were cross-sectional in nature, there was very little cross-validation of findings, 'hard' data such as physiological measures and archival records were used infrequently, and very few studies had combinations distinguishing design strengths such as multiple data sources and longitudinal observations.

The positivist paradigm is very dominant in North American organisational psychology, and the findings would be a little different if based upon research published in European journals. Also, adherents to the qualitative paradigm do not hold with all of Schaubroeck and Kuehn's implicit and explicit values concerning what constitutes good research.

Given the diversity of the roots and theoretical perspectives of organisational psychology, it is not surprising that many different tools are used for data collection (see Table 5.3).

Some organisational psychologists take a pragmatic approach and use the techniques that are most convenient and/or permitted by people in charge of the setting in which they are working. For reasons of philosophy (often expressed in terms of a favoured paradigm), other psychologists prefer some techniques over others and frame research questions which are suited to them. There is a considerable literature on the development of validated instruments (questionnaires) to measure psychological dimensions (see Box 5.2).

Quantitative data collected by advocates of the positivist paradigm are often subjected to complex statistical analyses. For example, Rousseau and Tijoriwala (1999) demonstrated how organisational psychologists use quantitative data to investigate quite complex sets of beliefs and perceptions and link them with theory – in this case it was nurses' beliefs about reasons for change in ward management techniques. This is particularly the case in non-randomised studies where statistics are used to compensate for an absence of controlled conditions. For example, groups of research participants may be compared using multifactorial analyses of variance, often with multiple dependent variables (outcomes) as well as independent variables (predictors). Control variables are included and specific hypothesised interaction effects are tested. The impact of a range of independent variables on a dependent variable is often tested using multiple regression techniques employing theoretically driven rationales to select the order which independent variables are entered into the regression equation. Statistical checks have to be performed for multi-collinearity (i.e. overly high correlations) between independent variables, and for the excessive influence of outlying data points. Structural equation modelling (SEM) is now quite commonly used to test the goodness-of-fit of the data collected with proposed theoretical models. SEM uses multiple indicators of variables to derive latent variables, which consist of observed data stripped of

Table 5.3 Some data-collection tools used in organisational psychology

Data collection tool	Description
Self-report questionnaire	Usually in paper form, but increasingly presented electronically. Poses respondents with a number of questions which can concern subjective and/or objective matters. Responses may be closed (e.g. agree/disagree) or open, where the respondents write what they see fit.
Other-report questionnaire	As above, but here somebody is providing information about somebody else, e.g. perceptions of their personality.
Psychometric test	Again, usually paper or electronically based, this aims to assess aspects of people's abilities or personality.
Structured interview	A face-to-face or telephone/teleconference interaction where the researcher puts a predetermined set of questions to a respondent or group of respondents.
Semi-structured interview	As above, but the set of questions includes a core asked to all respondents, and others that are either not specified in advance, or are specified, but only asked if it seems useful.
Unstructured interview	Here there is little predetermined other than a general topic area to explore with the respondent(s), going in directions that seem appropriate and will probably differ between respondents.
Structured qualitative instrument	Respondents are asked to write responses to open-ended questions, or to complete unfinished sentences, and their responses are then scored, classified or interpreted according to a predetermined template.
Repertory grid	An instrument where respondents specify or are presented with a number of stimuli (elements) (e.g. people they know) and are then invited to identify dimensions (constructs) upon which the elements may differ or be similar.
Observation of behaviour	The behaviour of people participating in research is directly observed and recorded. The researcher may do this overtly or covertly, and as a participant or detached observer.
Psychophysiological assessment	Biochemical or other data drawn from, for example, blood samples or monitoring of electrical activity in the brain.
Work output measures	Data concerning the quantity or, more rarely, quality of a person's work performance. These may be derived from verifiable information about productivity, or from performance ratings by others (see 'Other-report questionnaire' above).
Archival and personnel records	Data obtained from files or other information sources concerning, for example, employee absence, company profitability

Box 5.2 Development of a questionnaire to assess the climate for innovation

The Team Climate Inventory (TCI) was developed to assess the extent to which the climate in a work team was conducive to innovation. This work was part of a broader study of innovation in management teams in the National Health Service in Britain. Anderson and West (1998) used existing theory to suggest four facets of innovation that might be applicable to work teams – vision, participative safety, task orientation, and support for innovation. They devised sixty-one questions based on these four areas and collected data from 243 individuals in twenty-seven senior management teams. The statistical technique called factor analysis was used to identify the dimensions underlying the responses, and it was found that five distinct dimensions were present. Several of these bore a strong resemblance to the four facets of innovation identified from theory. A suitably amended set of questions was then tried out on a new sample of 971 people, including senior managers, primary care workers and oil company teams. The factor structure of these data was tested for consistency with the five-factor model using confirmatory factor analysis. A final version of the TCI was produced, containing thirty-eight questions assessing five aspects of innovative climate.

Although the primary aim was to describe the development of the TCI, it also showed that the climate for innovation in senior management teams was stronger than in primary health care teams, especially regarding vision and support for innovation. Senior managers also scored somewhat higher on those two factors than a sample of oil company teams. This is a good example of how organisational psychologists attempt to develop self-report measures that are designed to approximate an objective reality, and which can be used to diagnose aspects of current operating strengths and weaknesses, perhaps as a basis for working on the latter.

error variance. It then estimates path coefficients between the latent variables, and provides a range of indicators of goodness-of-fit in order to indicate how plausible the proposed causal model is given the data obtained (see Box 5.3).

Proponents of the qualitative paradigm may use content analysis, where

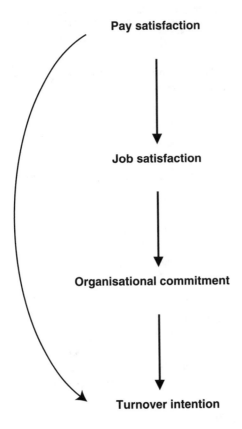

Pay satisfaction

Job satisfaction

Organisational commitment

Turnover intention

Figure 5.1 Model of turnover intent of nurses

Source: Lum *et al.* 1998

people's responses, or parts of them, are categorised according to the theme(s) evident in what they say or write. For example, Rosenthal *et al.* (1996) interviewed male and female health service managers about occasions

Box 5.3 Impact of pay policies on nurse turnover

Lum and colleagues (1998) obtained data from 361 nurses in an American teaching hospital. Established questionnaires were utilised to assess constructs that appear in a lot of organisational psychology research – namely organisational commitment, pay satisfaction, job satisfaction and turnover intention. They used structural equation modelling to test several possible causal models involving these variables. The model they derived from the data is shown in Figure 5.1.

In this model, pay satisfaction has both a direct effect on turnover intention and an indirect one through job satisfaction and organisational commitment. However, pay satisfaction explains only about 4 per cent of the variance in turnover intention, which, although highly significant statistically, is not a very big effect in practical terms, especially when one considers that there is still a missing link at each end of the causal chain – from pay level/rise to pay satisfaction, and from turnover intention to actual turnover.

(Lum *et al.* 1998)

when they performed well or badly at work, and coded the qualitative data according the attributions used to explain the successes and failures. Often, but not always, evidence is presented concerning the reliability of the analysis. To determine reliability, another researcher categorises the data, and the frequency with which their categorisation agrees with that of the first researcher is calculated (see Box 5.4).

Box 5.4 Theories of innovation

A study using qualitative methods to test theory was reported by King (1992). He worked for two periods of approximately one month each as a nursing assistant on a psychogeriatric ward in a large district general hospital. Clinical staff there knew he was conducting research, so his role as participant observer was explicit. King's aim was to document the sequence of events surrounding innovations that were proposed for how the ward should operate – these were often quite small things but, nevertheless, new and a discernible change to the status quo.

Altogether he documented seven innovation histories. He also took two prominent theories of the innovation process and described each using six statements. He then asked two psychologists with no knowledge of the specific theories being tested to indicate whether each statement was applicable to each innovation. He discovered that one theory was more reliable in the sense that the

> two raters agreed in most of their judgements about its applicability, but that the other theory was more valid in the sense that it was more often rated as applicable to the innovation histories documented by King. He discussed his findings partly in terms of their implications for how the successful introduction of innovations can be managed and guided by theory.
>
> (King 1992)

There are, of course, many other ways of analysing textual or spoken data other than content analysis (see Chapter 3 in this volume) (Symon and Cassell 1998). For example, attributional analysis concerns the ways people account for the causes of events. Discourse analysis involves interpretation of the linguistic and rhetorical techniques people use to provide convincing accounts in specific contexts (see Box 5.5). This is much more holistic than content analysis, and is part of an attempt by the organisational psychologist to offer their own account of the (often conflicting) themes and purposes embedded in spoken and written material, and of how people construct their worlds through language.

Box 5.5 Rationale for British general practitioners to apply for fundholding status

As part of a study that included other (non-health service) groups, Cohen and Musson (2000) examined the use of entrepreneurial discourses in competition with other discourses by eighteen British general practitioners involved in an innovative way of funding their practices (fundholding). The authors defined 'discourse' as reflecting individuals' systematic use of language to articulate personal, collective and institutional meanings and values. They pointed out that there were often alternative discourses available that become more openly in competition with each other during times of change.

The GPs were interviewed, and also more informal 'coffee-table' chat was noted. The researchers discerned three rationales for applying for fundholding status: financial viability, autonomy for the practice, and better service for patients. Decisions about activities which were paid for by the government tended to be explained in terms of a business discourse, even though many of the GPs articulated a medical discourse in discussing other topics.

(Cohen and Musson 2000)

Limitations

Organisational psychology is not as well geared as organisational sociology to the identification of macro-social influences on individual behaviour, although there are some recent and notable exceptions. (Patterson *et al.* 1997). Psychologists tend to be more aware of individuals, groups, and the proximal influences on them. Organisational psychologists are interested in many organisation-wide variables such as 'downsizing' (reducing the size and staff numbers of an organisation), but primarily in terms of their impact on individuals rather than what they say about, for example, who wields power. Hence broader social issues of power, social and economic events and history tend to be neglected, though needless to say there are exceptions (Brotherton 1999).

On the whole, organisational psychologists do not expect to calculate the monetary value or cost of behavioural variables or management interventions such as the adoption of teamworking or the promotion of a particular organisational culture. Linked to this, along with many other people, most organisational psychologists would have trouble giving unequivocal answers to questions about cost-effectiveness – for example, what is the most efficient promotion policy? Yet even here there are exceptions. Utility analysis has been applied to the use of selection techniques with known validities in order to calculate the cash value, in terms of improved performance and/or reduced turnover, of adopting them in any given organisation (Raju *et al.* 1990).

Other potential limitations depend on one's point of view. Some would argue that any research where those who provide data are aware that they are doing so is likely to be compromised because the very awareness changes responses. Laboratory experiments are often criticised because the artificiality of the situation may well induce untypical behaviour. Any self-reported data may fail to get at the real reasons for people's behaviour, if Nisbett and Wilson (1977) are correct in their conclusion that we are unable to report these things accurately even when motivated to do so. Even apparently objective data drawn from records are likely to be incomplete and/or inaccurate, as many psychologists who have tried to obtain information about employee absence or turnover (for example) know only too well. In the current context, the most obvious limitation is that the efficiency or effectiveness of health service delivery is rarely the outcome of interest.

Perhaps, though, the limitations are more to do with the gap between the methods potentially available and those actually used in some organisational psychology research. Limitations on researchers' time, and restrictions on what managers in an organisation being researched will permit, contribute to this gap. Schaubroeck and Kuehn's findings notwithstanding, many papers *submitted* to organisational psychology journals (not necessarily published) use entirely cross-sectional quantitative self-report data on a largish (150+) non-random sample with a low response rate. Hypotheses are often rather arbitrarily derived from theory, and sometimes more attention is paid to the statistical significance of the findings than to their practical importance. Although they are often perhaps not as compelling or as far-reaching as one would hope, there are, thankfully, usually some useful practical implications to the findings.

Further reading

Arnold, J., Cooper, C. and Robertson, I. (1998) *Work Psychology*, 3rd edn, London: FT Pitman Publishing.

Breakwell, G. M., Hammond, S. and Fife-Schaw, C. (1995) *Research Methods in Psychology*, London: Sage.

Cook, T. D. and Campbell, D. T. (1979) *Quasi-experimentation: Design and Analysis Issues for Field Settings*, Chicago: Rand McNally.

Hesketh, B. (1993) 'Measurement issues in industrial and organizational psychology', in C. L. Cooper and I. T Robertson (eds) *International Review of Industrial and Organizational Psychology*, vol. 8, Chichester: Wiley.

Judd, C. M., McClelland, G. H. and Culhane, S. E. (1995) 'Data-analysis: continuing issues in the everyday analysis of psychological data', *Annual Review of Psychology*, 46: 433–65.

Symon, G. and Cassell, C. (eds) (1998) *Qualitative Methods and Analysis in Organizational Research: a Practical Guide*, London: Sage.

References

Anastasi, A. (1988) *Psychological Testing*, 6th edn, New York: Macmillan.

Anderson, N. and West, M. (1998) 'Measuring climate for work group innovation: development and validation of the team climate inventory', *Journal of Organizational Behavior*, 19: 235–58.

Arthur, M. B. and Rousseau, D. M. (eds) (1996) *The Boundaryless Career*, Oxford: Oxford University Press.

Brotherton, C. (1999) *Social Psychology and Management*, Buckingham: Open University Press.

Cohen, L. and Musson, G. (2000) 'Entrepreneurial identities: reflections from two case studies', *Organization*, 7: 31–48.

Hemingway, M. A. and Smith, C. S. (1999) 'Organizational climate and occupational stressors as predictors of withdrawal behaviours and injuries in nurses', *Journal of Occupational and Organizational Psychology*, 72: 285–300.

James, L. R. and James, L. A. (1989) 'Causal modelling in organizational research', in C. L. Cooper and I. T. Robertson (eds) *International Review of Industrial and Organizational Psychology*, vol. 4, Chichester: Wiley.

King, N. (1992) 'Modelling the innovation process: an empirical comparison of approaches', *Journal of Occupational and Organizational Psychology*, 65: 89–100.

Lum, L., Kervin, J., Clark, K., Reid, F. and Sirola, W. (1998) 'Explaining nursing turnover and intent: job satisfaction, pay satisfaction, or organizational commitment?', *Journal of Organizational Behavior*, 19: 305–20.

Nisbett, R. E. and Wilson, T. D. (1977) 'Telling more than we can know: verbal reports on mental processes', *Psychological Review*, 84: 231–59.

Patterson, M., West, M., Lawthom, R. and Nickell, S. (1997) *Impact of People Management Practices on Business Performance*, London: Institute of Personnel and Development.

Raju, N. S., Burke, M. J. and Normand, J. (1990) 'A new approach for utility analysis', *Journal of Applied Psychology*, 75: 3–12.

Rosenthal, P., Guest, D. and Peccei, R. (1996) 'Gender differences in managers' causal explanations for their work performance: a study in two organizations', *Journal of Occupational and Organizational Psychology*, 69: 145–52.

Rousseau, D. M. and Tijoriwala, S. A. (1999) 'What's a good reason to change? Motivated reasoning and social accounts in promoting organizational change', *Journal of Applied Psychology*, 84: 514–28.

Schaubroeck, J. and Kuehn, K. (1992) 'Research design in industrial and organizational psychology', in C. L. Cooper and I. T Robertson (eds) *International Review of Industrial and Organizational Psychology*, vol. 7, Chichester: Wiley.

Swanson, V., Power, K. and Simpson, R. (1998) 'Occupational stress and family life: a comparison of male and female doctors', *Journal of Occupational and Organizational Psychology*, 71: 237–60.

Symon, G. and Cassell, C. (eds) (1998) *Qualitative Methods and Analysis in Organizational Research: a Practical Guide*, London: Sage

Taber, T. D. (1991) 'Triangulating job attitudes with interpretive and positivist measurement methods', *Personnel Psychology*, 44: 577–600.

Chapter 6

Policy analysis

Stephen Harrison

Introduction

The varied approaches to policy analysis and the wide range of literature
and techniques on which its practitioners draw, make it impractical to offer
either a stipulative definition or a consensual account. The characterisation
of policy analysis presented here is broadly consistent with several classic
texts, most notably Jenkins (1978), Hogwood and Gunn (1984) and Parsons
(1995). Policy analysis contains three central ingredients: the policy making
process, its context, and the use and development of theory.

Definition and theoretical basis

Policy analysis is less a well defined method than a general approach to
issues in public policy, famously described as an 'art and craft' (Wildavsky
1980). Some of its roots are in political science (a discipline which, apart
from psephology, is notoriously pragmatic methodologically). From this it
inherits the assumption that the social world is occupied by actors with
different and sometimes conflicting interests, and with differences in power
relative to each other, and that institutional arrangements (such as government and organisations) are important mediators of the outcomes of these
differences. Other important roots of policy analysis are in the more technical discipline of operations research, in which mainly quantitative
methods are employed to optimise a specified function (see Chapter 10), but
it is fair to say that any social science might contribute. If 'government' is
taken to include local public agencies, a useful definition of the focus of
policy analysis is 'what governments do, why they do it, and what difference
it makes' (Heidenheimer *et al.* 1990: 3); thus 'policy' does not necessarily
mean 'high policy' and policy analysis can certainly be employed at the level
of local health care organisations, implying some overlap of subject matter
with organisational studies (see Chapter 2).

First, 'policy' is conceived of as a *process*, rather than simply as an output
of a decision or an input to management. Such a process is regarded as

including several stages (for an alternative view, see Sabatier and Jenkins-Smith [1993]), such as:

- agenda setting
- defining what is thought to be problematic and what objectives would represent an acceptable improvement
- elucidating the causal structure of the problem
- elucidating measures that would intervene in this causal structure
- appraising the options for intervention
- implementation of selected options
- evaluation and feedback.

Policy analysts are often reluctant to make assumptions about logic or rationality. Despite their resemblance to 'rational-comprehensive' decision theory, the stages set out above are not assumed to be sequential, nor even necessarily present in respect of any particular policy, and the behaviour (as well as the intentions) of relevant actors is of interest, as are unintended consequences (such as perverse incentives), inaction, non-decisions, symbolic action and *post facto* rationalisations. An important strand of policy analysis is concerned with decision making, and there is a long tradition of retrospective studies of disastrous decisions about public policy (see for example Janis [1972] on the 'Bay of Pigs', and Gouran *et al.* [1986] on the *Challenger* space shuttle disaster). Thus policy analysts are well aware, for instance, that policies may go on while the problem to which they are supposed to be a solution changes, or while policy makers decide that it is the solution to a completely different problem. The history of community care is a good example of the latter: originally a therapeutic model, it became a solution to the problems of long-stay institutions and subsequently a cost-saving device.

Second, action is seen as taking place within a *context* which both affects and may be affected by the policy process. The nature of relevant context will vary with the policy area, and perhaps with the macro or micro level of the subject studied. In health policy, it is likely to include considerations such as current and changing political, economic and social climates, demographics and contemporary technological developments (Harrison and Moran 2000). At a more micro level, factors such as (multi-) organisational and professional cultures, organisational resources, and competing policy agendas will be relevant (Harrison 1994a).

Third, policy analysis is concerned with the use and development of explicit *theory*, not just the assembly of data nor the attribution of causes without an understanding of causal process. The assumption here is that all discussion of (actually or potentially) causal processes is theory-laden; hence the only choice is between treating theory implicitly or explicitly. The arguments in favour of the latter were neatly summed up many years ago by J. M. Keynes:

> Practical men, who believe themselves to be quite exempt from any intellectual influences, are usually the slaves of some defunct economist.
>
> (Keynes 1936: 383)

In other words, making theory explicit permits, and indeed encourages us to question the taken-for-granted: to consider, for instance, whether our facts could be interpreted in other ways, or whether our assumptions are out of date (for a discussion, see Harrison *et al.* [1990: 3–6]). It is important to be clear that 'theory' is not necessarily 'grand' or overarching theory; in common with organisation studies (see Chapter 2), policy analysis is typically concerned with what have been referred to as 'theories of the middle range' (Merton 1968). In epistemological terms, policy analysts tend to espouse some version of realism, though this does not exclude the recognition that, for instance 'problems' and 'acceptable solutions' are socially constructed (Murphy *et al.* 1998; Hammersley 1992) (see Chapter 1); they therefore make a pragmatic distinction between 'fact' and 'value' while recognising that these become closely intertwined in policy analysis, along with theory. Analysis of an issue might typically include:

- *values* – what state of affairs is unsatisfactory? What means of addressing the problem would be acceptable? (means are subject to value judgements as well as ends)
- *facts* – for whom is it unsatisfactory and how do different actors 'frame' the problem? Which actors would find which solutions acceptable? How is the incidence of the problem distributed? How is it changing and how quickly?
- *theories* – what has caused the problem and what interventions would improve matters?

Uses

In broad terms, the foci of policy analysis can be divided into two overlapping clusters of concerns (Hill 1997). Though the balance may vary, common to both clusters is the recognition of policy as process that occurs in context and is best understood with the aid of explicit theory. Also common to both is the notion of the stages of the policy process outlined above; it is not the case that the clusters refer to different segments of that process. One cluster, which Parsons (1995) has labelled 'analysis of the policy process', is very much related to some of the traditional concerns of political science, that is the development of detailed descriptions of the policy process in specific cases and of theoretically informed explanations of its operation more generally. It might thus overlap with the interests of historians and biographers (see Chapter 9) and with the more critical wing of organisation studies (see Chapter 2), being concerned with understanding, for instance:

- how issues come to be seen as problematic and how they come to be defined in particular terms rather than others (Hogwood and Gunn 1984)
- how issues reach policy agendas and why others do not (Kingdon 1984)
- how policies and decisions are made, and what options are rejected
- the (normative and explanatory) theories espoused by relevant actors (Young 1977)
- the effect of implementation attempts on the policy itself
- why (on occasions irrespective of their apparent effects) policies survive or are abandoned

It can readily be seen that studies in this first cluster may be unwelcome to policy makers (a term which is employed throughout this chapter to include senior managers), since their findings may not correspond to the level of achievement claimed for policies, may attribute less effect to the leadership of individuals than those individuals might desire, might stress symbolic rather than practical politics (Edelman 1977), and indeed might show that cherished policies came about accidentally (Harrison 1994b).

The second cluster, which Parsons (1995) has labelled 'analysis in and for the policy process', centres on problem solving and policy or programme evaluation, that is on defining problems and plausible solutions, and on learning what programme interventions 'work' in what conditions. The latter will often be *social programmes*: those that aim to change the behaviour of social groups, whether staff in the relevant programmes or their recipients/users. Studies within this cluster may be more obviously normative than in the other cluster, and may sometimes commence from the policy maker's own perspective of the problem, especially if the analysis is undertaken by commissioned consultants or an in-house policy unit. In keeping with the influence of political science, the approach may also be attractive in the evaluation of programmes with multiple stakeholders with different perspectives and interests (Smith and Cantley 1985). However, other studies may be more explanatory; policy analysts may well evaluate programmes devised by others and see their work adding to a body of social scientific knowledge. A key consideration for policy analysts working on this second cluster of concerns is that they are usually unable to manipulate the policy or its implementation in a way that would allow the use of experimental research designs. Some of the consequences of this are discussed in the next section.

There is a growing demand in many countries for policy analysis of a kind that falls within the second cluster of concerns described above. This chapter, therefore, concerns itself only with these aspects of policy analysis. This is not to imply that policy analyses falling within the first cluster of concerns would not be worthwhile (Harrison 1998), or that the results of studies falling within the second cluster will always be welcomed (or used) by policy makers.

How to undertake policy analysis

It follows from the above characterisation of policy analysis, as a potentially multidisciplinary approach to a wide range of questions about national and local policy and its implementation, that it is neither possible nor appropriate to present a prescriptive step-by-step account of 'how to do it'. What follows is therefore an outline of some of the methods that policy analysts might use, and the kinds of questions they need to ask of themselves, their clients (where appropriate) and their data. As noted above, this exposition relates only to the second cluster of policy analysts' concerns outlined. For presentational purposes, this cluster can be further subdivided into two types of study; it should be emphasised, however, that these are not wholly distinct. The first refers to the analysis of policy from the starting point of a particular perceived problem, whereas the second begins from a potential solution that has been implemented.

Analysing policy problems

Where analysis commences from a situation that is perceived to be a problem by policy makers or other relevant stakeholders, the following basic data are likely to be required.

- Which actors perceive what situation to be problematic? How much agreement is there about this?
- Why is the situation seen to be problematic? (For example, what values does it violate? What pressure is being applied to policy makers by other actors who consider it problematic?)
- In what terms is the problem 'framed' by various actors? (For example, is it seen as an economic, or political, or legal, or moral problem?)
- What facts are taken to constitute evidence of the perceived problem? Upon whom do these facts impact? What is the prevalence of the problem, and how is it changing? Is it all really the 'same' problem?
- What measures have been posited as plausible solutions to the problem? To which actors are such measures acceptable and unacceptable?
- What evidence exists about the effectiveness or otherwise of posited solutions to the problems? How valid and relevant is this evidence, and how applicable is it to the context in which the perceived problem has been identified?

A number of features and consequences of this approach require further comment. First, it can be noted that the underlying academic discipline of political science is clearly manifest in the emphasis placed on differences in actors' values and perspectives.

Second, it should be noted that actors are as likely to have values about the *means* of securing policy ends as about the ends themselves; thus policies may be technically effective but (say) politically unacceptable.

Third, some rigorous questioning of the context of reported facts may be necessary in order to establish whether they bear out the apparent nature of the problem. To take some examples, it is clear that 'the unemployed' include people in very different situations (between jobs, seeking the first job, waiting to start training), as do 'patients' (the otherwise well but acutely ill, otherwise well on long-term medicine, those in hospital, those requiring palliative care, etc.). When it comes to examining policy solutions, these groups may well need to be disaggregated.

Fourth, the assessment of the plausibility of solutions, and of evidence about their effectiveness, requires a serious attempt to understand the causal structure of the problem (Hogwood and Gunn 1984) as perceived by relevant actors. One approach to this is to attempt to elicit their theories about the problem and posited solutions, and to build them into a rough model. A worked example of such a rough model is provided in Figure 6.1 and Box 6.1.

Box 6.1 Theory of teenage pregnancy

This model shows the (explicit and implicit) theoretical assumptions made in a report on teenage pregnancy. This model is an attempt to map in a reasonably systematic fashion someone else's knowledge and assumptions about a particular problem. Such models are not equivalent to the 'path-analytic' diagrams sometimes found in social scientists' quantitative analyses and which attempt to show the relative weights of contribution to an outcome made by different variables. Rather, this model focuses on process and can be used to clarify and examine the inherent plausibility of assumed causal structures of the problems. Models such as this can be used to relate espoused theories to an existing body of evidence, to compare rival 'framings' of problems, and to clarify the relationships of actual or proposed policy interventions to assumed causal structures. It should be clear that such models contain only a rather coarse notion of causality, and although they are theoretical, they cannot really be thought of as fully developed theories.

(Social Exclusion Unit 1999)

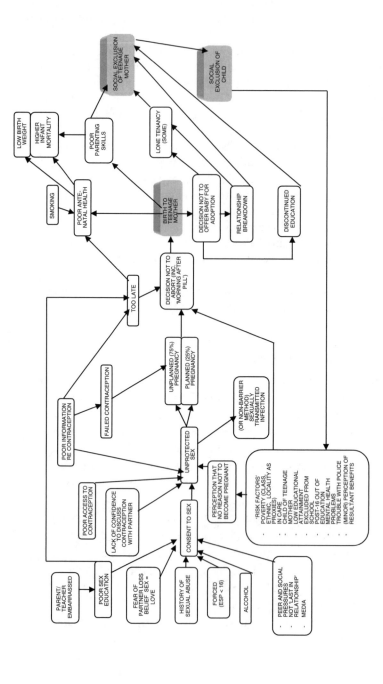

Figure 6.1 An implied theory of teenage pregnancy based on Cm4342, 1999

Source: Author's interpretation of Social Exclusion Unit 1999

Note: Health Warning! The purpose of this figure is to illustrate a mode of policy analysis rather than to offer an authoritative account of teenage pregnancy: see text.

A contrasting approach is to build a logical 'ideal type' model in order to identify the circumstances in which a posited solution might be effective. A worked example is provided in Box 6.2, drawing on the work of Gunn

---

Box 6.2 Gunn's conditions for 'perfect implementation' adapted for 'evidence-based medicine'

1   That there are sufficient material resources *in the appropriate combination* available.
2   That there are sufficient non-material resources available.
3   That the policy to be implemented is based upon a valid theory of cause and effect.
4   That the relationship between cause and effect is direct and that there are few, if any, intervening links.
5   That external dependency relations are minimal.
6   Either:

•   that the necessary tasks are fully specified in correct sequence (implying that policies should be capable of reduction to a detailed set of instructions) *and* the implementers have the power to impose their wishes

or:

•   that there is understanding of, and agreement on objectives of the policy and how they are to be implemented, throughout the implementing organisation; that is, that there should be no conflicts within the implementing organisation and that everyone should clearly understand what they have to do and when.

Condition 1 reminds us that the question of resources goes beyond money: plentiful funds may not be able to overcome (say) skills or drugs shortages and there must be no supply 'bottlenecks'.

Condition 2 reminds us that time is a non-trivial factor, since members of real-world organisations have ongoing activities and other priorities with which new policies have to compete for attention.

Condition 3 draws our attention to the need for research (and perhaps justifies the current level of rhetoric about 'evidence-based policy').

Condition 4 reminds us that most organisational endeavours require the cooperation of teams of individuals, and that the more links in the chain, the more likely it is that at least one will break

down. If we imagine each individual to have an independent probability of cooperation, the total probability of perfect implementation
will be the product of all the individual probabilities; only ten links
each with a (high) probability of 0.95 produces a total probability of
0.57, little better than evens! Of course, such probabilities in the real
world are unlikely to be independent, since individuals are influenced
by the behaviour of colleagues. Thus this condition also serves to
remind us of the importance of organisational 'culture'.

Condition 5 refers to political factors such as the refusal of other
organisations to cooperate in implementing the policy, and the same
mathematical considerations apply as above.

Finally, condition 6 reminds us that organisations are frequently
characterised by resistance, conflict, disagreement and misunder-
standing.

(adapted from Harrison 1994a, after Gunn 1978)

(1978). It addresses the question of how 'evidence-based medicine' might
effectively be implemented by setting up an ideal model of 'perfect implementation', which is unlikely ever to be achieved in practice but which draws
attention to factors that would-be implementers need to address.

The types of empirical data that are needed in order to undertake policy
analysis are clearly rather varied. Data about policy makers' beliefs, perceptions and theories may be obtained from secondary sources such as
speeches, media reports, manifestos and policy documents, or from primary
sources such as interviews and autobiographies. Data about the empirical
manifestation of the perceived problem may be available from routine official sources, but it is an obvious possibility that the purposes for which such
data and classifications are originally designed may render them less than
adequate for subsequent policy analysis. Moreover, the linkage of data from
different sources about individuals may be inhibited by ethical considerations. If a specific matter has come to be seen as an issue or problem, the
actors who perceive it as such may have collected data as part of their
campaign and may make it available to policy analysts, though of course the
latter will be aware of the possibility that such data have been selected in
order to underpin a particular 'framing' of the issue. The collection of ad
hoc data about a problem may therefore be preferable, but is clearly dependent on resources, available timescale and the willingness and ability of

public agencies to respond conscientiously to surveys and other data requests.

Less descriptive evidence about the perceived problem, its causes and plausible policy solutions may be obtained from published academic sources, though 'grey' literature such as local case studies or student dissertations may be a significant source in some cases. Major difficulties exist in systematically reviewing and aggregating such material (see Chapter 12). First, it may simply be hard to find, since unless the topic is highly technical it can be difficult to determine appropriate search terms for electronic databases. Thus journals may have to be hand-searched, and written requests for 'grey' literature sent to relevant university departments and public agencies. There may be relevant material from rather different policy or organisational contexts. Second, the matter of how such material might be summarised or aggregated is not straightforward, given that it is likely to include studies employing a variety of methods in a variety of contexts. It is certainly desirable to conduct a review of such material in a way that it is transparent and systematic, but the techniques of systematic review and meta-analysis that have become conventional in health technology assessment are unlikely to be practicable; even if such techniques were practicable, the focus of policy analysis on trying to understand *process* would militate against exclusive reliance on 'black box' methods (i.e. methods which focus on outcomes instead of processes). One answer to these problems of aggregation and subsequent generalisation is to regard the evidence as a potential contribution to theory development (Pawson and Tilley 1997), a matter to which the next subsection returns.

Evaluating policy interventions

Research topics in the field of health service delivery and organisation will often possess two characteristics. First, they are intimately concerned with *social* processes and technologies; that is, they imply attempts to modify the behaviour of either staff or patients. Second, these processes and technologies are *diffuse* in the sense that they are not single or simple variables (see Box 6.3).

Box 6.3 Evaluating business process re-engineering in a hospital

Packwood and colleagues (1998) discuss the applicability to hospitals of business process re-engineering (BPR), a recent approach to improving organisational performance.

BPR is defined as 'the fundamental rethinking and radical redesign of business processes to achieve dramatic improvements in critical, contemporary measures of performance, such as cost, quality, service and speed' (Hammer and Champy 1993).

This is a good example of a research topic concerned with social processes, where changes in behaviour of staff are central. Moreover, the broad scope of BPR means that it is very diffuse. After a general discussion of BPR and the public sector, the authors introduce a case study of an individual hospital in London where the technique was used. It was found to be a matter of contention among participants whether BPR had been successful in their hospital. Changes in attitude of staff were found to have been as important as behaviour: staff were more open to change and had been given some tools for its management. If that were to lead to improved behaviour, it would be difficult to identify a precise cause and effect. The study also shows the importance of exploring in detail the processes actually undertaken under a term such as 'BPR', as these are likely to vary considerably from one organisation to another, depending on local circumstances.

(Packwood et al. 1998)

An increasingly prominent area of political emphasis is upon 'joined-up thinking' and multi-agency working as the means of addressing complex health and social problems. Figure 6.1 showed the breathtaking complexity and diffuseness of just one area, teenage pregnancy.

It follows that the investigation of these matters by the randomised trials conventionally employed in health technology assessment may be unable to provide policy prescriptions, and that the second cluster of policy-analytic tools outlined above has a clear potential role in researching health service delivery and organisation (defining problems and plausible solutions, and learning what programmes 'work' in what conditions [see Box 6.4]).

Box 6.4 Evaluating stroke units

'Stroke unit' is a term used to denote a system of organised inpatient care which aims to reduce mortality and long-term institutionalisation after stroke. The concept is therefore not one which is well defined, but perhaps the key element is that it is distinguished from what is assumed to be the more usual form of care for such patients, that is on a general medical ward. The diffuseness of such a technology presents a number of obvious problems for evaluation by means of a randomised trial.

First, given the broad definition of the intervention, it is hard for evaluators to be confident that they are aggregating like with like, whether in the context of a primary study or a systematic review or meta-analysis. Thus stroke units in different hospitals may differ from each other in respect of various policies, such as: how long after the stroke event the patient may be admitted; how long the patient may remain in the unit; the discreteness of physical location; the composition of the clinical team; and the actual micro-level clinical interventions employed.

Second, if studies were to show that stroke units reduced mortality and/or dependency, as seems to be the case (Langhorne et al. 1993; Stroke Unit Trialists' Collaboration 1997), the policy consequences would be uncertain: how would one 'roll out' such a technology?

Third, since the technology is to a considerable extent social, it is likely that explanations of its outcome will need to take into account matters of organisational and wider culture, details of which are unlikely to have been collected in randomised trials and would be hard to reproduce in a 'roll-out'.

Researchers working within the tradition of randomised trials have sought to address the first and (to some extent) the second of these issues by retrospectively interviewing trialists about the characteristics of the stroke units studied in their original primary research, showing that there is a good deal of homogeneity in their characteristics and that many of these are much less likely to be found in other settings for stroke care (Stroke Unit Trialists' Collaboration 1997). Nevertheless, the basic problem remains; policy prescriptions for social interventions require causal explanations couched in terms of process. The approaches to the analysis of policy problems and interventions offer a purchase on this problem.

The approaches described above are all likely to be useful as preparatory stages for an empirical study aimed at evaluating the impact of a specific policy intervention. However, some further considerations of study design arise when a topic is approached from this direction. As noted, policy analysts are rarely able to manipulate variables or allocate (randomly or otherwise) research subjects, implying that other means of establishing validity, assigning attribution and identifying counterfactuals need to be developed. Comparative case studies (sometimes thought of as 'natural experiments') are seen as an especially important means to this end. The adequacy of the 'controls' provided by comparative case studies will depend on what cases are available and how the policy analyst is able to assemble them into a structure of meaningful comparisons. Thus, if the policy intervention to be evaluated has been universally implemented, the comparisons can only focus on different *contexts* of implementation, perhaps (if thought to be of potential significance) comparing urban with rural, large with small, or client group with client group. It should be noted that there is little reason to structure comparisons around factors for which there is neither existing evidence nor plausible *a priori* reasoning concerning an effect on the impact of the policy. If a policy intervention has not been universally imposed, the possibility arises for comparisons between cases of implementation and non-implementation (see Chapter 4), or of differential forms of implementation. Indeed, it may even be possible to construct comparisons which utilise both types of comparison, providing the structure illustrated in Figure 6.2, a sort of quasi-Latin square design to help distinguish the impact of policies from that of changing environments and for helping to attribute the contribution of particular variables.

Despite these devices, policy analysts are often reluctant to claim that social research can be authoritative. The reasons for this are well established in the social science literature, and have been aptly summarised by Pawson and Tilley (1997). In the context of *social* change, causation can only be understood:

- as part of the social relations and organisational structures in which it is embedded
- as a product of interaction between agency (the reasoning and choices that individuals make) and structure (their capacity to put these into action)

	Large organisation	Small organisation
Intervention adopted	Case A	Case B
Intervention not adopted	Case C	Case D

Figure 6.2 Two-dimensional controls through comparative case studies

Note: The dimensions of comparison are arbitrary examples: see text

- as occurring only contingently, that is, in the context of favourable social rules, norms, and values
- as occurring within an already self-transforming social system

Recognition of this has led policy analysts in two rather different directions. One has been to argue that research and analysis should be seen as an aid to the development of interactive solutions to problems, that is to identify the perspectives of the various stakeholders (Smith and Cantley 1985), and to help them to conceptualise or reconceptualise the problem and to negotiate (implicitly or explicitly) mutually acceptable solutions (Lindblom and Cohen 1979). The other direction has been to seek ways of generalising from *case study* data (see Chapter 2), arguing that general conclusions can be drawn from multiple or even single case studies, so long as data about context, processes and policy outcomes are conscientiously collected and adequately analysed (Yin 1994). These considerations, alongside policy analysts' interest in process, their realist epistemology, and their inability to manipulate variables or research subjects, has made 'scientific realism' an attractive approach to the 'what works?' questions within the policy analytic process (Pawson and Tilley 1997; Sayer 1984). The axiom of this approach is to provide causal social explanations in the form 'outcomes result from mechanisms acting in context'. The implication of such an approach is that generalisation of research findings cannot take place through aggregation, but rather through the *development of theory*. In Pawson and Tilley's own words (1997: 116):

> Cumulation is a matter of deepening, specifying, focusing and formalising our understanding of program [*sic*] mechanisms, contexts and outcome patterns … a matter of traversing between general theory … and empirical case studies.

This is unlike generalisation based on population sampling, which Pawson and Tilley (1997) argue to be inappropriate for programme evaluation on the grounds that there are so many elements of programme, institutions and context that:

> the very notion of the 'representativeness' or 'typicality' of a case gets lost as the descriptive baselines increase … [thus] generalisation is not a matter of understanding the *typicality* of a program in terms of its routine conduct. Rather the process of generalisation is … one of *abstraction*. We move from one case to another not because *they* are descriptively similar but because *we* have ideas that can encompass them both.

This corresponds to long-standing social scientific ideas of 'analytical induction', an analytic process which includes iteration between data and theory, with refinement or rejection of the latter dependent on negative instances or deviant cases (Yin 1994; Mason 1996; Murphy *et al.* 1998) (see also Chapter 1).

Limitations

I have given an account of policy analysis which focuses on both its core assumptions and the topics which it is designed to address. I have also stressed that policy analysis is not a single set of closely related techniques, but rather an orientation towards addressing these kinds of topics. Within these parameters, the limitations of policy analysis are, perhaps ironically, political rather than technical. These political limitations can be roughly divided into two groups.

One group of limitations relates to the attitudes of what might be termed the health services academy, which in recent years has been marked by a hardening orthodoxy (perhaps symbolised by references to *the* 'hierarchy of evidence' [Harrison 1998]) in favour of the view that valid causal knowledge is best derived from studies which utilise randomised controlled trials. This hardening of academic opinion has been matched by the creation of research programmes and of academic departments premised on that opinion. Policy analysts have to work hard for a place in this structure.

The second group of political limitations relates to the potential response of policy makers to policy analysis, and has been identified by Hogwood and Gunn (1984: 263–8). Analysis may suggest that particular problems are intractable or that there are no 'quick fixes'; analysis may expose uncomfortable differences between the values of different stakeholders; analysis may explicate matters in a way that makes political 'fudges' (and hence consensual decisions) more difficult. All of this is neatly encapsulated in the title of the American edition of Wildavsky's (1980) classic text on policy analysis, *Speaking Truth to Power*. Yet if political aspirations for open government and participatory democracy are to be realised, these limitations represent a price to be paid.

Further reading

Hill, M. (1997) *The Policy Process in the Modern State*, London: Prentice Hall.

Hogwood, B. W. and Gunn, L. A. (1984) *Policy Analysis for the Real World*, Oxford: Oxford University Press.

Murphy, E., Dingwall, R., Greatbatch, D., Parker, S. and Watson, P. (1998) 'Qualitative research methods in health technology assessment: a review of the literature', *Health Technology Assessment*, 2, 16: 1–272.

Parsons, W. (1995) *Public Policy: an Introduction to the Theory and Practice of Policy Analysis*, Aldershot: Edward Elgar.

Pawson, R. D. and Tilley, N. (1997) *Realistic Evaluation*, London: Sage.

Yin, R. (1994) *Case Study Research: Design and Methods*, Thousand Oaks CA: Sage.

References

Edelman, M. (1977) *Political Language: Words that Succeed and Policies that Fail*, New York: Institute for the Study of Poverty.

Gouran, S. D., Hirokawa, R. Y. and Martz, A. E. (1986) 'A critical analysis of factors related to decisional processes involved in the Challenger disaster', in B. R. Patton, K. Giffin and E. N. Patton (eds) *Decision Making Group Interaction*, New York: Harper and Row.

Gunn, L. (1978) 'Why is implementation so difficult?', *Management in Government*, 33, 4: 169–76.

Hammer, M. and Champy, J. (1993) *Re-engineering the corporation: a manifesto for business revolution*, London: Harper Collins.

Hammersley, M. (1992) *What's Wrong With Ethnography?*, London: Routledge.

Harrison, S. (1994a) 'Knowledge into practice; what's the problem?', *Journal of Management in Medicine*, 8, 2: 9–16.

——(1994b) *Managing the National Health Service in the 1980s: Policy Making on the Hoof?*, Aldershot: Avebury.

——(1998) 'The politics of evidence-based medicine in the UK', *Policy and Politics*, 26, 1: 15–32.

Harrison, S., Hunter, D. J. and Pollitt, C. (1990) *The Dynamics of British Health Policy*, London: Unwin Hyman.

Harrison, S. and Moran, M. (2000) 'Resources and rationing: managing supply and demand in health care', in G. L. Albrecht, R. Fitzpatrick and S. C. Scrimshaw (eds) *The Handbook of Social Studies in Health and Medicine*, 493–508, London: Sage.

Heidenheimer, A. (1986) 'Politics, policy and polizey as concepts in English and continental languages: an attempt to explain divergences', *Review of Politics*, 48, 1: 3–30.

Heidenheimer A., Heclo, H. and Adams, C. T. (1990) *Comparative Public Policy: the Politics of Social Choice in America, Europe and Japan*, 3rd edn, New York: St Martin's Press.

Hill, M. (1997) *The Policy Process in the Modern State*, London: Prentice Hall.

Hogwood, B. W. and Gunn, L. A. (1984) *Policy Analysis for the Real World*, Oxford: Oxford University Press.

Janis, I. L. (1972) *Groupthink: Psychological Studies of Policy Decisions and Fiascoes*, Boston MA: Houghton Mifflin.

Jenkins, W. I. (1978) *Policy Analysis*, Oxford: Martin Robertson.

Keynes, J. M. (1936) *The General Theory of Employment, Interest and Money*, London: Macmillan.

Kingdon, J. W. (1984) *Agendas, Alternatives and Public Policy*, Boston MA: Little, Brown.

Langhorne, P., Williams, B. O., Gilchrist, W. and Howie, K. (1993) 'Do stroke units save lives?', *Lancet*, 342: 395–8.

Lindblom, C. E. and Cohen, D. K. (1979) *Usable Knowledge: Social Science and Social Problem Solving*, New Haven: Yale University Press.

Mason, J. (1996) *Qualitative Researching*, London: Sage.

Merton, R. K. (1968) *Social Theory and Social Structure*, New York: Free Press.

Murphy, E., Dingwall, R., Greatbatch, D., Parker, S. and Watson, P. (1998) 'Qualitative research methods in health technology assessment: a review of the literature', *Health Technology Assessment*, 2, 16: 1–272.

Packwood, T., Pollitt, C. and Roberts, S. (1998) 'Good Medicine? A case study of business process re-engineering in a hospital', *Policy and Politics*, 26, 4: 401–15.

Parsons, W. (1995) *Public Policy: an Introduction to the Theory and Practice of Policy Analysis*, Aldershot: Edward Elgar.

Pawson, R. D. and Tilley, N. (1997) *Realistic Evaluation*, London: Sage.

Sabatier, P. A. and Jenkins-Smith, H. C. (eds) (1993) *Policy Change and Learning: An Advocacy Coalition Approach*, Boulder: Westview Press.

Sayer, A. (1984) *Method in Social Science: A Realist Approach*, London: Hutchinson.

Smith, G. and Cantley, C. (1985) *Assessing Health Care: A Study in Organisational Design*, Milton Keynes: Open University Press.

Social Exclusion Unit (1999) *Teenage Pregnancy*, Cm4342, London: Social Exclusion Unit.

Stroke Unit Trialists' Collaboration (1997) 'Collaborative systematic review of the randomised trials of organised inpatient (stroke unit) care after stroke', *British Medical Journal*, 314: 1151–9.

Wildavsky, A. (1980) *The Art and Craft of Policy Analysis*, London: Macmillan.

Yin, R. (1994) *Case Study Research: Design and Methods*, Thousand Oaks CA: Sage.

Young, K. (1977) 'Values in the policy process', *Policy and Politics*, 5, 2: 1–22.

Chapter 7

Economic evaluation

Mark Sculpher

Introduction

This chapter considers the role of economic evaluation in studying the delivery and organisation of health services. First, economic evaluation is defined and its theoretical foundations explained; then the uses of economic evaluation are considered; next an account of how to undertake economic evaluation, with some examples of recent studies, is provided; and finally, some limitations of economic evaluation in this area are discussed.

Definition and theoretical basis

Economic evaluation is a set of analytic tools to assess the value for money of alternative ways of allocating limited resources to health care. Formally defined, it is 'the comparative analysis of alternative courses of action in terms of both their costs and their consequences' (Drummond *et al.* 1997). Aspects of this definition need to be emphasised. The first is that economic evaluation is comparative; in other words, it is only possible to comment on the value for money of a programme or intervention in comparison to another. The second point to note is that economic evaluation is focused on both resource effects (costs) *and* non-resource consequences which include every impact that is potentially of value to users and potential users (e.g. health effects, convenience, access, etc.).

The theoretical foundations of economic evaluation lie in welfare economics, the area of economics concerned with the normative question of how to assess whether one state of the world (i.e. allocation of resources) is preferable to another (Boadway and Bruce 1984). This contrasts with the aim of organisational economics, which is designed to describe and to understand behaviour (see Chapter 8). The dominant paradigm in welfare economics has been the neoclassical movement, and in particular the work of Pareto (Blaug 1985). The cornerstone of Paretian welfare economics is the normative value judgement that a movement from one state of the world to another (i.e. a reallocation of resources) is justified if at least one person is made better off and nobody is made worse off. Logically, therefore, allocative efficiency is defined as a state of the world when nobody can be made better off without somebody being made worse off.

Economic theory has explored the extent to which the free market can be seen as a vehicle for allocating scarce resources in a manner consistent with the neoclassical concept of allocative efficiency (Gravelle and Rees 1992). However, an important area of theoretical and applied research in the post-war period has been devoted to the use of economic analysis, based on the principles of Paretian welfare economics, in allocating resources where a free market is limited or absent, such as in health care. In this context, the weakness of the Paretian value judgement for policy analysis resulted in the concept of the *potential* Pareto improvement (Boadway and Bruce 1984). This criterion justifies a change from one state of the world to another if the gainers from the change could *potentially* compensate the losers and still remain better off overall. From an efficiency standpoint, the potential for such a change is sufficient; whether compensation is actually paid is an issue relating to the distribution of resources.

A set of applied analytic tools – cost-benefit analysis (CBA) – was born out of this fusion of welfare economic theory and the need to make policy decisions (Sugden and Williams 1979). Used widely to inform decision making relating to major infrastructure investments, CBA seeks to appraise alternative policy options in a way consistent with the potential Pareto improvement criterion. This is achieved by quantifying the benefits to gainers and the disbenefits to losers in the same units, usually in monetary terms. In other words, CBA is a set of quantitative methods to compare the costs and benefits of programmes, and a policy will be deemed efficient if the benefits outweigh the costs.

A range of theoretical issues has been raised in operationalising CBA in general, including how to value resources where no formal market exists (e.g. clean air), and how to aggregate across individuals whose valuation of different policy outcomes may differ largely because of inequality in income (Johanesson 1995). However, the fundamental characteristics of health care delivery in most developed countries – namely the rejection of a free market as the main mechanism for resource allocation and the major role of the public sector in finance and delivery – required formal analytical techniques to replace the market's 'free hand' in determining how resources should be allocated (Arrow 1963). Although some early attempts at CBA exist in the health care field (Schoenbaum *et al.* 1967), the use of these methods has been problematic. The main reason for this is the difficulty in valuing the outcomes of health services – in particular health effects but also a range of other valued effects such as convenience and information – on the same monetary scale as costs. Much of the early use of CBA in health assumed that the only valued outcome of health care programmes was increased economic productivity as a result of improved longevity and reduced morbidity. However, this was criticised and, in due course, rejected on the basis that changes in health (and other outcomes of health care programmes) are valued in their own right by individuals and that this should be reflected in economic evaluation methods (Mishan 1971).

Although CBA has retained a limited role in health care, largely as a result of the development of contingent valuation methods to value the effects of programmes in monetary terms (Gafni 1991), economic evaluation in the area has moved towards a separate set of analytical methods – cost-effectiveness analysis (CEA). Whereas CBA appeals to the Paretian concept of allocative efficiency, CEA focuses on a more limited concept of efficiency: technical efficiency, the maximisation of the outcomes of health care for a finite level of resources (Doubilet *et al.* 1986). CEA is rather easier to apply to health care than CBA because outcomes need not be valued in monetary terms. However, these methods introduce their own restrictions, in particular the need for outcomes to be valued on a single generic scale that facilitates comparison across disparate areas of health care activity.

Although attempts have been made to link CEA in health care with welfare economic theory (Garber *et al.* 1996), CEA has focused on health gain (or surrogates for this). This contrasts with traditional welfare economics where the implications of alternative programmes for individuals' utilities were its prime focus. This is given expression in CBA through individuals' willingness to pay for the attributes of those programmes which may include health and non-health effects. This dissonance between CEA and traditional welfare economics has led to the placement of much applied economic evaluation in health care into an 'extra-welfarist' theoretical framework which places less emphasis on individuals' utilities in social decision making and more emphasis on measurable health gain (Culyer 1989).

Uses of economic evaluation in health care

Most published economic evaluations relate to health care technologies such as therapeutic and diagnostic interventions, and screening programmes (Elixhauser *et al.* 1998). Establishing the value for money of pharmaceuticals is an area in which the methods have been increasingly applied over the last ten to twenty years, largely as a result of attempts, in various health care systems, to control the growth in the cost of new pharmaceutical interventions. However, the rationale for economic evaluation includes the appraisal of any change in health care resource allocation, including changes in the way services are delivered, models of care, organisational approaches and settings for care. In any health care system resources available for health care are limited. In the context of resource constraints, a series of economic questions can be addressed. For example:

- What will be the net cost implications of an open-access endoscopy service, led by nurse practitioners, compared to the existing physician referral-based system?
- What benefits and disbenefits would such a system have, relative to current practice?
- If the new system generates some additional benefits for patients but also has some limitations, how do we weigh up these advantages and disadvantages to arrive at an overall conclusion about whether or not the change leads to a net gain in benefit?
- If the new system costs more than existing practice, how do we assess whether those additional resources should be devoted to this new programme compared to other organisational initiatives and to new (more costly) therapeutic interventions (e.g. a new drug for Alzheimer's disease)?

These questions are central to the rationale of CEA, as shown in Figure 7.1.

Figure 7.1 shows the comparison of two forms of health care delivery – for example, open-access endoscopy (A) versus a standard referral-based system (B). To establish whether open access is more cost-effective than standard practice, the differential costs and benefits of the two forms of delivery need to be compared. If open access is shown to be less costly and to generate more benefits than standard practice (bottom right quadrant of Figure 7.1), it can be considered economically dominant and unequivocally more cost-effective. The converse is true if standard practice is less costly and more beneficial (top left quadrant). Many health care programmes will actually be placed in the top right quadrant – adding to costs but also improving benefits. Sometimes a new form of service delivery might have

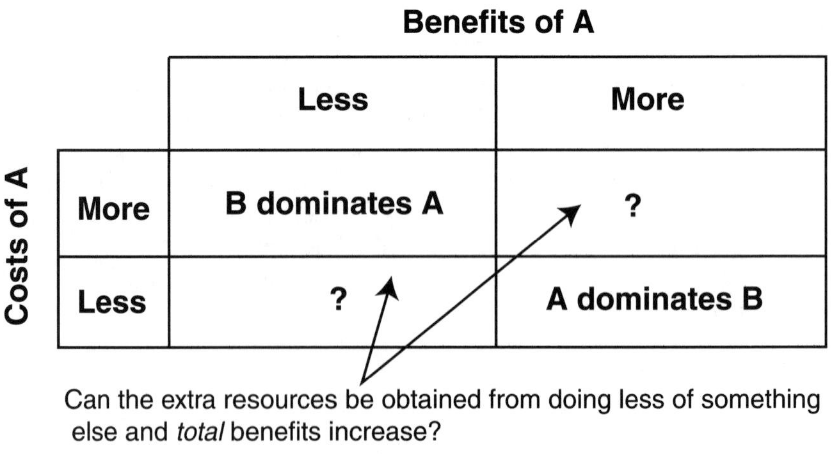

Benefits of A

		Less	More
More		B dominates A	↗ ?
Less		? ↗	A dominates B

Costs of A

Can the extra resources be obtained from doing less of something else and *total* benefits increase?

Figure 7.1 Assessing the cost-effectiveness of two interventions

some detrimental effects but reduce costs (bottom left quadrant). In this context, it is still possible for the new form of service delivery to be cost-effective. The key criterion – in the top right quadrant, for example – is whether the additional resources necessary to provide the new service can be 'freed up' elsewhere in the system and still generate a net gain in benefit. If the open-access endoscopy service was found to be more costly but more beneficial than existing arrangements, could, for example, fewer hernia repairs be undertaken to fund the change in delivery? The open-access scheme could be considered cost-effective if the net change in benefits as a result of doing fewer hernia repairs and introducing the open-access endoscopy service was positive.

How to undertake economic evaluation

Although the need formally to assess the value for money associated with potential changes in resource configuration is clear, as part of research on the delivery and organisation of services, this description of the principles of CEA raises a series of questions about how methods which have developed largely in the field of health technology assessment can be adapted for appraisal of delivery mechanisms and organisational arrangements.

Measurement of costs and benefits

A growing proportion of economic evaluation of health technologies is undertaken using data from randomised controlled trials (RCTs). In this context, data are collected prospectively on patient-specific resource use (e.g. days in hospital, drug consumption, physician visits) to facilitate an analysis of the differential cost of the interventions under comparison (Drummond and Davies 1991). The trial format also generates estimates of the differential impact of the interventions on factors other than resource use, which is the first stage in defining the benefit side of the CEA illustrated in Figure 7.1. However, it has been recognised that RCTs also have a number of disadvantages as a vehicle for economic evaluation, in particular the problems associated with limited external validity as a result of trials typically including atypical patients treated by unrepresentative clinicians in specialist centres, and the short-term follow-up of patients (Drummond 1994). For this reason, and because the use of randomised trials in the evaluation of many health care interventions is often difficult in practice, many economic evaluations use data taken from other sources such as non-randomised studies and patient surveys. Indeed, economic evaluation requires a range of data inputs, and some parameters – in particular the unit costs of particular resources – are appropriately taken from sources other than RCTs.

Decision analytic methods

Even if the data available are not ideal and there is considerable uncertainty about the costs and effects of different forms of service delivery, decisions need to be taken about appropriate resource allocation. The need to make decisions under conditions of uncertainty has resulted in decision analysis becoming a major element in the armamentarium of economic evaluation (Weinstein and Fineberg 1980; Sculpher *et al.* 1997). Decision analysis is a formal framework in which data from RCTs, non-randomised designs, and experts are carefully and rigorously elicited and formally synthesised to address the issue of cost-effectiveness. Decision analytic techniques have been used widely to evaluate screening programmes where, like many delivery and organisation issues, RCTs are often difficult to undertake successfully (see Box 7.1) (Eddy 1990; Ades *et al.* 1999). Decision analytic techniques have been used much less frequently in respect of service delivery and organisational issues themselves.

Box 7.1 Using decision analysis techniques to evaluate antenatal screening for HIV

Ades and colleagues (1999) used an incremental cost-effectiveness analysis, relating additional costs of screening to years of life gained, in order to assess the cost-effectiveness of universal antenatal HIV screening, compared to selective screening. A decision model was used to generate prevalence thresholds of undiagnosed HIV infection in pregnant women above which universal screening would be cost-effective. These thresholds were compared with estimates of prevalence of undiagnosed HIV infection in women in each UK health authority, in order to determine which health districts should adopt universal screening, and which districts should not, as prevalences there were too low for universal screening to be cost-effective.

The decision model was constructed using cost data concerning screening itself and the costs of care for both mother and child; benefit data concerning the years of life gained for the mother and child; and data concerning rates of vertical transmission of HIV infection from mother to child with and without the risk-reduction strategies which screening allows one to introduce.

The results showed that universal HIV antenatal screening would be cost-effective throughout the United Kingdom, as long as test costs were kept low and uptake of screening was high.

(Ades *et al.* 1999)

As a framework for conceptualising an economic evaluation, synthesising data and reaching a decision, it is possible to use decision analytic models to evaluate potential changes by

- characterising existing practice in terms of the process of care (resources used, management pathways for patients, impact on intermediate or health-related outcomes)
- identifying the scope for improvement in services and simulating how changes in organisation and delivery might impact on various types of outcome
- prioritising new data collection using primary research methods – this can involve valuing the additional information in monetary terms (Claxton 1998)
- on the basis of existing or new data, estimating the impact of policy changes on resources and various types of outcome, and estimating the cost-effectiveness of the change
- providing an indication of the uncertainty around the decision and hence indicating the priorities for yet further data collection

Perspective

Central to any economic evaluation is the issue of whose costs and benefits are to be considered. In principle, economic evaluation is concerned with the efficient use of all societal resources, and hence considers the use of resources other than those of the health services. As shown in Figure 7.2, a broad perspective on costs would include the resource implications of programmes for other parties, including public agencies (e.g. social services, education), employers and patients (e.g. travel costs, the value of time forgone consuming health services). Perspective is also important on the benefit side, and again an interest in societal efficiency would demand a broad view of benefit, extending beyond patients to include parties such as informal carers and the families of patients.

In relation to the appraisal of health technologies, the importance of a societal perspective has been emphasised in methodological guidelines (Gold *et al.* 1996). The issue of costs incurred by patients has been a particularly important area of research and debate in the economic evaluation field (Torgerson *et al.* 1994). Arguably, in the context of the economic evaluation of service delivery, a broad perspective on costs and benefits is particularly important. The study reported by Wooten *et al.* (2000) is an example of an evaluation of a mode of service delivery (telemedicine) where some attempt was made to include social costs, but this was not done fully. A better example of the importance of fully including social costs is given by Roberts *et al.* (1989) (in Box 7.2) where the costs and benefits of public health surveillance in respect of infected confectionery are demonstrated.

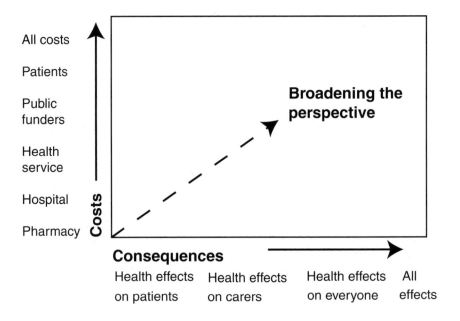

Figure 7.2 The perspective of an economic evaluation

The broad, societal perspective on costs and benefits is important because many potential changes will involve trade-offs between health service resources and patient costs. For example, research looking at the most appropriate location for a new health care facility will have to balance a potential reduction in the cost to the health service of a centralised facility in, say, a city centre, due to economies of scale, with the increased cost this may impose on patients in terms of travel and time. With an evaluation of this type, ignoring costs to patients would not be consistent with any consideration of societal efficiency. Furthermore, the costs patients face in

---

Box 7.2 An economic evaluation of public health surveillance including social costs

Roberts and colleagues (1989) reported a study which showed that the use of the public health surveillance system in England to identify and enable the prompt withdrawal of a consignment of chocolate contaminated with *Salmonella napoli* had significant economic benefits, when all costs were taken into account. These costs included the social costs, as well as the costs of investigation and testing and the

costs of health care. The latter two categories of costs were designated 'public sector costs'. The social costs were costs to families and
society, consisting of direct costs of illness to families; costs
attributable to loss of productive activity (mainly due to family
members not working when caring for the victims of the infection);
costs attributable to pain, suffering and death (including the value of
lives saved by the prompt withdrawal of the contaminated product);
and the costs to industry of withdrawing the product from sale. The
cost of the outbreak was over £500,000. It was estimated that five
deaths were prevented by the intervention and that 185 admissions
to hospital and 29,000 cases of S. napoli were avoided. The successful
investigation yielded a 3.5-fold rate of return to the public sector and
23.3-fold rate of return to society on an investment in the public
health surveillance system.

consuming health care represent 'access costs' which have been shown to
explain differential take-up of services (Acton 1975).

Valuing benefits

Programmes changing health outcomes

Measuring benefits in the evaluation of health care delivery poses some
particular (although not unique) problems. CEA in health care has moved
towards a focus on relating resource use to the health gain associated with
interventions. Although this has had the advantage of avoiding the monetary valuation of outcomes that is required for CBA, the process of
measuring and valuing health for CEA is controversial.

The controversy centres around the fact that health is undoubtedly multidimensional – a characteristic that is reflected in the use of
multidimensional measures of health status such as the SF-36 (Ware and
Donald Sherbourne 1992). However, CEA requires that the benefits of
health care are expressed on a single-dimensional scale that facilitates an
assessment of which of the programmes under comparison generates the
greatest benefit overall, and the extent of that additional benefit. The focus
of research has been on the use of preferences to weight different outcomes
onto a single metric that also has a generic quality that facilitates comparison across treatment areas and specialities. A range of techniques has
emerged from this research, including contingent valuation (for use in CBA)
(Gafni 1991) and healthy-year equivalents (Mehrez and Gafni 1991).
However, from the viewpoint of applied CEA, by far the most frequently

used generic measure of benefit has been the quality-adjusted life year (QALY) (Weinstein and Stason 1977). The QALY combines patient longevity and individuals' preferences about different levels of health-related quality of life into a single measure which, in principle, has meaning across all areas of health service activity (Torrance and Feeny 1989). Although the QALY is based on a number of strong assumptions about individuals' preferences and has remained a source of controversy (Loomes and McKenzie 1989), it has been used as 'an index of health' in CEA in many health care systems (Tengs *et al.* 1995).

How useful will the QALY be in the economic evaluation of service delivery? Much depends on what the aim is. Some changes in the organisation and delivery of services are aimed at improving patients' health. For example, an objective of delivering cancer care in specialised centres is the improvement of patients' prognoses by concentrating quality services (staff, equipment) and ensuring high levels of throughput to maintain and develop professionals' skills. Other changes are more focused on freeing up resources (health service and other) without a detrimental effect on patients' health (see Box 7.3). Changes in delivery to make services more convenient to patients is an example of where the aim is to release patients' resources (i.e. time). Although the focus is the efficient use of resources, efficiency can only be assessed if the implications of health outcomes are considered. If positive or negative effects on patients' health seem plausible, it is important to express benefits using available measures of health suitable for CEA, such as QALYs.

Box 7.3 Cost analysis of hospital-at-home

A cost analysis of hospital-at-home compared to standard in-patient care of orthopaedic patients found costs per day were lower for the hospital-at-home scheme, but the durations of orthopaedic episodes (i.e. care in the hospital and at home) were longer, making total costs for hospital-at-home higher than for standard inpatient care.

(Hensher et al. 1996)

Table 7.1 shows some recent examples of economic evaluations of the way services are delivered and organised.

It can be seen from these studies that there is a focus on health outcomes, which have been measured in various ways, though none of the studies considered the impact of changes in terms of QALYs. This may have been prompted in some studies (e.g. open-access follow-up for inflammatory bowel disease) by the fact that the analysis showed economic dominance:

Table 7.1 Examples of economic evaluations

Intervention	Benefits	Design
Community leg ulcer clinics (Morrell *et al.* 1998)	• Ulcer healing • Satisfaction	Randomised controlled trial
Referrals facilitator in mental health (Grant *et al.* 2000)	• Psychological well being • Social support	Randomised controlled trial
GP versus nurse practitioners (*Venning et al.* 2000)	• Process (e.g. length of consultation) • Satisfaction • Generic health status	Randomised controlled trial
Open-access follow-up for inflammatory bowel disease (Williams *et al.* 2000)	• Generic health status • Disease-specific health status	Randomised controlled trial

one option being less costly and no less effective than its comparators. In other studies, where an intervention was shown to be more costly and more beneficial (e.g. the referrals facilitator), it may have been considered that it would not have been possible to register the clinical gains shown in the study in terms of QALYs. However, for these organisational developments, it will not be possible to use formal analysis to establish that the additional benefits are greater or less than could be achieved if additional resources were devoted to another development or a new (or the expansion of a) health technology.

It is likely that making the link between service organisation and delivery and impact on health will not be an easy research objective – randomised trials, for example, would probably need to include large numbers of patients followed up over many years to quantify the link (see Chapter 4). However, this is also a feature of the relationship between many health technologies and health gain. This is particularly the case with diagnostic technologies (Severens and van der Wilt 1999). In this context, decision modelling has much to offer as a framework for economic evaluation, synthesising available data from a range of sources to make the link between organisational factors and health-related outcomes. See Box 7.4 relating to the economic evaluation of implementation interventions.

The use of decision analysis and of QALYs as a specific way of representing health benefits takes an aggregated approach to economic

> **Box 7.4 Evaluating implementation strategies**
>
> Implementation strategies are interventions designed to alter health professionals' behaviour in a manner consistent with good research evidence. Most primary research – including both randomised trials and non-randomised studies – has focused on establishing a link between implementation strategies, such as computer prompts and audit, and changes in process characteristics such as the proportion of practice reflecting the evidence-based guidelines. To the extent that implementation strategies result in an increase in costs, the cost-effectiveness of their use can only be assessed by establishing a link to health gain (Mason et al. 1999). This is because the ultimate objective is to improve health; because a huge range of new and established health technologies, as well as organisational aspects, will be competing for resources with the implementation strategies, so a comparison of their benefits using a common metric is essential. Decision modelling offers a way of linking evidence on the effectiveness of implementation strategies, in terms of process changes in professional behaviour, with longer-term changes in health outcomes and costs using available evidence on the costs and benefits of the interventions that the implementation interventions are seeking to encourage.
>
> (Sculpher 2000)

evaluation. In other words, these sorts of methods are used to synthesise available evidence, together with assumptions and relevant preferences, to provide an explicit framework for identifying an optimal solution to a particular problem. However, this approach to economic evaluation has its opponents, with some arguing that economic evaluation should be focused on describing the costs and effects of interventions and programmes, leaving the incorporation of preferences and assumptions to decision makers (Freemantle and Mason 1999). This contrast between implicit decision making by decision makers and explicit use of analytical techniques has not been informed by empirical research on the approach that generates the best decisions.

Programmes with effects other than on health

Some organisational arrangements will not have the objective of effecting health outcomes. Rather, they will be focused on non-health attributes of services that are of value, such as information provision, speed of delivery and quality of relationship with health care professionals. A recent major study looking at the costs and benefits of a picture archiving and communications system (PACS), used a range of non-randomised methods including time series analysis (Bryan *et al.* 2000). This study is discussed in more detail in Chapter 4.

Alternatively or additionally, benefits for staff in terms of, for example, job satisfaction may be the focus. There has been some debate about whether these 'process attributes' of health care should be considered to be distinct from health outcomes in economic evaluation (Ryan and Shackley 1995). Economic evaluation ideally needs to be able to value process attributes using the same metric as for health gain.

The QALY has limitations in this context, as available methods for generating its preference weights focus on changes in health; there are no examples of process attributes being incorporated into the QALY. One possibility is the use of conjoint analysis, which is an approach to valuation that was developed largely outside health care in areas such as marketing and environmental evaluation (Ryan and Farrar 2000). Recently it has been used to evaluate a range of health services, including examples of changes in service delivery, such as time spent on a waiting list (see Box 7.5), blood transfusion support and patient health cards.

Box 7.5 Use of conjoint analysis techniques

Ryan and Farrar (2000) illustrated how conjoint analysis techniques could be used in a study of the trade-offs that individuals were willing to make between location of treatment and waiting time in the provision of orthodontic services. Patients attending three orthodontic clinics in Scotland were asked to make choices between two alternatives in fifteen scenarios. The characteristics used in the scenarios concerned the location of the first and second orthodontic appointment (hospital or local clinic in each case) and the waiting time (twelve or sixteen months). Results indicated that patients were willing to wait an extra 1.3 months to have their first appointment at a local clinic.

(Ryan and Farrar 2000)

A common approach to conjoint analysis in the health care field is discrete choice analysis that involves a series of steps.

1   Selecting a series of attributes which are likely to be affected by a programme. These attributes can be process-related or health-related.
2   Divide these attributes into levels.
3   Present a choice of scenarios to a sample of individuals of interest (e.g. patients, members of the public) where each scenario represents a combination of attributes at different levels, and ask respondents to indicate their preferred scenario.
4   Present further choices between scenarios where each choice involves changes to one or more of the levels of the attributes.

The appropriate analysis of responses provides an indication of individuals' preferences over the attributes of interest. In particular, discrete choice analysis can show how respondents trade off the various attributes. For example, in the study described in Box 7.5 it is possible to explore the trade-offs that individuals were willing to make between location of treatment and waiting time for orthodontic services.

The role of conjoint analysis in economic evaluation has yet to be fully established. If one of the attributes presented is the cost imposed directly on the respondent, then trade-offs between attributes can be expressed in monetary terms. For example, it would be possible to estimate the average amount respondents were willing to pay for a particular gain in health or change in process attributes. With money as the metric, conjoint analysis could generate measures of benefit for use in CBA to compare different service configurations. As yet it is not clear whether conjoint analysis can offer a route to non-monetary generic measures of benefit for CEA.

Limitations

Economic evaluation is limited to assessing the efficiency of the delivery of health services. To improve its contribution, there are a number of methodological issues that would benefit from further research. These include the development of modelling techniques to make the link between changes in service delivery and the impact on health, where this is the objective of the change. Further development of methods is needed for valuing process attributes on a single scale suitable for use in economic evaluation and using a scale where health itself is an attribute, to show trade-offs between process and health attributes.

Economic evaluation would also benefit from the strengthening of analyses of non-randomised data in an attempt to reduce bias, and enhancement of modelling and other techniques to generalise from studies undertaken in specific centres and locations to routine practice.

Further reading

Drummond, M. F., O'Brien, B. J., Stoddart, G. L. and Torrance, G. W. (1997) *Methods for the Economic Evaluation of Health Care Programmes*, New York: Oxford University Press.

Gold, M. R., Siegel, J. E., Russell, L. B. and Weinstein, M. C. (1996) *Cost-Effectiveness Analysis in Health and Medicine*, New York: Oxford University Press.

Patrick, D. L. and Erickson, P. (1993) *Health Status and Health Policy. Allocating Resources to Health Care*, New York: Oxford University Press.

Weinstein, M. C. and Fineberg, H. V. (1980) *Clinical Decision Analysis*, Philadelphia: W. B. Saunders.

References

Acton, J. P. (1975) 'Nonmonetary factors in the demand for medical services: some empirical evidence', *Journal of Political Economy*, 83: 595–614.

Ades, A. E., Sculpher, M. J., Gibb, D. M., Gupta, R. and Ratcliffe, J. (1999) 'A cost-effectiveness analysis of antenatal HIV screening in the UK', *British Medical Journal*, 319: 1230–4.

Arrow, K. J. (1963) 'Uncertainty and the economics of medical care', *American Economic Review*, 53: 91–6.

Blaug, M. (1985) *Economic Theory in Retrospect*, Cambridge: Cambridge University Press.

Boadway, R. W. and Bruce, N. (1984) *Welfare Economics*, Oxford: Blackwell.

Bryan, S., Buxton, M. and Brenna, E. (2000) 'Estimating the impact of a diffuse technology on the running costs of a hospital: a case study of a picture archiving and communication system', *International Journal of Technology Assessment in Health Care*, 16: 787–98.

Claxton, K. (1998) 'Bayesian approaches to the value of information: implications for the regulation of new pharmaceuticals', *Health Economics Letters*, 2: 22–8.

Culyer, A. J. (1989) 'The normative economics of health care finance and provision', *Oxford Review of Economic Policy*, 5: 34–58.

Doubilet, P., Weinstein, M. C. and McNeil, B. J. (1986) 'Use and misuse of the term "cost effective" in medicine', *New England Journal of Medicine*, 314: 253–6.

Drummond, M. (1994) *Economic Analysis Alongside Controlled Trials: An Introduction for Clinical Researchers*, Leeds: Department of Health.

Drummond, M. F. and Davies, L. (1991) 'Economic analysis alongside clinical trials', *International Journal of Technology Assessment in Health Care*, 7: 561–73.

Drummond, M. F., O'Brien, B. J., Stoddart, G. L. and Torrance, G. (1997) *Methods for the Economic Evaluation of Health Care Programmes*, New York: Oxford University Press.

Eddy, D. M. (1990) 'Screening for cervical cancer', *Annals of Internal Medicine*, 113, 3: 214–26.

Elixhauser, A., Halpern, M., Schmier, J. and Luce, B. R. (1998) 'Health care CBD and CEA from 1991 to 1996: an updated bibliography', *Medical Care*, 36: MS1–MS9.

Freemantle, N. and Mason, J. (1999) 'Not playing with a full DEC: why development and evaluation committee methods for appraising new drugs may be inadequate', *British Medical Journal*, 318: 1480–2.

Gafni, A. (1991) 'Willingness to pay as a measure of benefits', *Medical Care*, vol. 29: 1246–52.

Garber, A. M., Weinstein, M. C., Torrance, G. W. and Kamlet, M. S. (1996) 'Theoretical foundations of cost-effectiveness analysis', in M. R. Gold, J. E. Siegel, L. B. Russell and M. C. Weinstein (eds) *Cost-Effectiveness in Health and Medicine*, New York: Oxford University Press.

Gold, M. R., Siegel, J. E., Russell, L. B. and Weinstein, M. C. (eds) (1996) *Cost-Effectiveness in Health and Medicine*, New York: Oxford University Press.

Grant, C., Goodenough, T., Harvey, I. and Hine, C. (2000) 'A randomised controlled trial and economic evaluation of a referrals facilitator between primary care and the voluntary sector', *British Medical Journal*, 320: 419–23.

Gravelle, H. and Rees, R. (1992) *Microeconomics*, London: Longman.

Hensher, M., Fulop, N., Hood, S. and Ujah, S. (1996) 'Does hospital-at-home make economic sense? Early discharge versus standard care for orthopaedic patients', *Journal of the Royal Society of Medicine*, 89: 548–51.

Johanesson, P. O. (1995) *Evaluating Health Risks*, Cambridge: Cambridge University Press.

Loomes, G. and McKenzie, L. (1989) 'The use of QALYs in health care decision making', *Social Science and Medicine*, 28: 299–308.

Mason, J., Wood, J. and Freemantle, N. (1999) 'Designing evaluations of interventions to change professional practice', *Journal of Health Services Research and Policy*, 4, 106–11.

Mehrez, A. and Gafni, A. (1991) 'The health-years equivalent: how to measure them using standard gamble approach', *Medical Decision Making*, 11: 140–6.

Mishan, E. J. (1971) 'Evaluation of life and limb: a theoretical approach', *Journal of Political Economy*, 79: 687–705.

Morrell, C. J., Walters, S. J. and Dixon, S. (1998) 'Cost effectiveness of community leg ulcer clinics: randomised controlled trial', *British Medical Journal*, 316: 1487–91.

Roberts, J. A., Sockett, P. and Gill, O. (1989) 'Economic impact of a nationwide outbreak of salmonellosis: cost benefit of early intervention', *British Medical Journal*, 298: 1227–30.

Ryan, M. and Farrar, S. (2000) 'Using conjoint analysis to elicit preferences for health care', *British Medical Journal*, 320: 1530–3.

Ryan, M. and Shackley, P. (1995) 'Viewpoint: assessing the benefits of health care: how far should we go?', *Quality in Health Care*, 4: 207–13.

Schoenbaum, S. C., Hyde, J. N., Bartoshesky, L. and Krampton, K. (1967) 'Benefit–cost analysis of rubella vaccination policy', *New England Journal of Medicine*, vol. 294.

Sculpher, M. J. (2000) 'Evaluating the cost-effectiveness of interventions designed to increase the utilisation of evidence-based guidelines', *Family Practice*, 17: S26–S31.

Sculpher, M. J., Drummond, M. F. and Buxton, M. J. (1997) 'The iterative use of economic evaluation as part of the process of health technology assessment', *Journal of Health Services Research and Policy*, 2: 26–30.

Severens, J. L. and van der Wilt, G.-J. (1999) 'Economic evaluation of diagnostic tests: a review of published studies', *International Journal of Technology Assessment in Health Care*, 15: 480–96.

Sugden, R. and Williams, A. H. (1979) *The Principles of Practical Cost–Benefit Analysis*, Oxford: Oxford University Press.

Tengs, T. O., Adams, M. E., Pliskin, J. S., Safran, D. G., Siegel, J. E., Weinstein, M. C. and Graham, J. D. S. O. (1995) 'Five hundred life-saving interventions and their cost-effectiveness', *Risk Analysis*, 15: 369–90.

Torgerson, D. J., Donaldson, C. and Reid, D. M. (1994) 'Private versus social opportunity cost of time: valuing time in the demand for health care', *Health Economics*, 3: 149–55.

Torrance, G. W. and Feeny, D. (1989) 'Utilities and quality-adjusted life years', *International Journal of Technology Assessment in Health Care*, 5, 559–75.

Venning, P., Durie, A., Roland, M., Roberts, C. and Leese, B. (2000) 'Randomised controlled trial comparing cost-effectiveness of general practitioners and nurse practitioners in primary care', *British Medical Journal*, 320: 1048–53.

Ware, J. E. and Donald Sherbourne, C. (1992) 'The MOS 36-item short form health survey (SF36). 1. Conceptual framework and item selection', *Medical Care*, 30: 473–83.

Weinstein, M. C. and Fineberg, H. V. (1980) *Clinical Decision Analysis*, Philadelphia: W.B. Saunders.

Weinstein, M. C. and Stason, W. B. (1977) 'Foundations of cost-effectiveness analysis for health and medical practices', *The New England Journal of Medicine*, 296: 716–21.

Williams, J. G., Cheung, W. Y., Russell, I. T., Cohen, D. R., Longo, M. and Lervy, B. (2000) 'Open access follow up for inflammatory bowel disease: pragmatic randomised controlled trial and cost-effectiveness study', *British Medical Journal*, 320: 544–8.

Wooten, R., Bloomer, S., Corbett, R., Eedy, D., Hicks, H., Lotery, H., Mathews, C., Paisley, J., Steele, K. and Loane, M. (2000) 'Multicentre randomised control trial comparing real time teledermatology with conventional outpatient dermatology care: societal cost-benefit analysis', *British Medical Journal*, 320: 1252–6.

Chapter 8

Organisational economics

Diane Dawson

Introduction

Organisational economics is a term loosely used to encompass discussion of organisational behaviour emerging from research in a variety of disciplines including economics, management science, and business studies (Barney and Hesterly 1996). This chapter focuses on the contribution of economics to our understanding of the performance of organisations.

In recent decades there has been significant growth in the volume of research undertaken by economists on the organisation and delivery of health care services (Culyer and Newhouse 2000). The framework of analysis and the methods used are those employed in most other areas of applied microeconomics. The approach can best be understood by considering the questions asked, the concepts used and the research techniques employed.

Definition and theoretical basis

In 1932 Robbins provided a succinct statement of the objects of economic inquiry when he defined economics as the study of the allocation of scarce resources between competing ends. Later he elaborated on this basic definition when he referred to the subject matter of economics as those aspects of behaviour which in some way or another arise from the existence of scarcity (Robbins 1984). This concentration on the particular problems created by scarcity means that the issues examined by economists often appear narrow. Individuals and institutions are multifaceted, but the economist attempts to focus on one aspect of observed behaviour: factors influencing how individuals and institutions allocate scarce resources, and what changes in the environment might lead them to change the allocation. The research questions of economics concern the efficiency and equity of our arrangements for the management of scarcity. As the problems of accommodating rising expectations of health care within limited resources have become more serious and more public, it is not surprising that economics, as a discipline focused on how societies deal with scarcity, has played a larger role in health services research.

Given that the central questions of economic research are concerned with how scarcity is managed, *opportunity cost* is the central concept of cost used in economic analysis. If you cannot do everything, the cost of what you choose to do is having to accept that some other highly desirable outcome will now be forfeit. This leads to two other concepts central to all economic analysis. If agents cannot undertake all desirable activities, they must make choices and we will observe *trade-offs*. If a hospital manager decides to focus available new resources on development of cancer services, it will not be possible to proceed with a number of important improvements in orthopaedics. The rate at which treatments for cancer patients are traded off against orthopaedic treatments for other patients will be influenced by the resources required to provide both kinds of treatment, and by the objectives of the individuals making these decisions. This highlights the final key concept in all economic analysis, and that is the *margin*. The decision to focus extra resources on development of cancer services does not mean the hospital decides to cease providing orthopaedic treatments. There is some expansion of cancer services and a slight reduction in orthopaedics. Economic decisions focus on the margins of activity; trade-offs are at the margin. Consequently the key concept of cost becomes the *marginal opportunity cost* of any decision on resource use.

The structure of what is commonly referred to as the *neo-classical* model reflects the underlying scarcity problem. People are postulated to seek to maximise objectives, subject to the constraints they face. In applied work, interest often focuses on the effects of changing the constraints or the objects of choice. Introduction of new products or new technologies may extend the field of choice, and changes in budgets, input prices or introduction of a new regulation will alter the constraints. All such changes create incentives for individuals to change their behaviour.

Methodology, and especially epistemology, are not topics frequently discussed by applied economists. There is, as in most disciplines, a small minority who recognise the importance of methodological issues and, as in other areas of the social sciences, there are disputes over the most appropriate methods for economists to adopt for applied work in general and for research into the provision of health care in particular (Coast 1999; Mannion and Small 1999). The current position of mainstream economic research has been described as logical empiricism, a 'more cautious and moderate' form of logical positivism (Caldwell 1982) (see Chapter 1 for a discussion of positivism). The objective is to explain, not to merely describe and predict. Solow (1997) points out that the research questions of the vast majority of economists are policy-driven and data-driven rather than theory-driven.

As in all scientific endeavours, there is an important distinction to be drawn between normative and positive analysis. Within economics, normative analysis ordinarily relates to 'what should be' from an ethical or policy perspective, and positive analysis to actual behaviour or 'what happens' in practice. Effective policy cannot be designed or implemented without an appreciation of how agents and institutions behave, so both types of analysis are necessary. The contribution of normative analysis (economic evaluation) has been discussed in Chapter 7. This chapter focuses on positive analysis – research into behaviour. It is of course impossible to draw a clear line between the two, as the characteristics of the system chosen for positive study are often chosen because of their expected policy relevance. Implementation of policy itself affects behaviour (see Chapter 6). One of the better known laws of economics, Goodhart's Law, states that 'any observed statistical regularity will tend to collapse once pressure is placed on it for control purposes' (Goodhart 1984). While originally formulated in the context of monetary policy, it has important implications for the behaviour of organisations in the health care sector.

New Institutional Economics and its application to the organisation of health services

The majority of health economists use an analytic framework derived from neo-classical microeconomic theory, often now extended by developments in New Institutional Economics (NIE). Arrow (1963) in a paper many consider to have provided the research agenda for what he called the medical care industry, stressed the overwhelming importance of uncertainty in understanding organisation and performance in health care. New Institutional Economics takes as its starting point that societies develop institutions and organisations that serve to reduce the costs of allocating resources when people have different objectives, incomplete information and especially asymmetric information. It is therefore a particularly suitable framework for the analysis of organisations for the delivery of health care.

Modern health care requires management of diverse human and physical resources, and organisation of these activities is not costless. One of the earliest research questions of NIE was investigation of the conditions under which costs of organising production of a good or service would be reduced if two organisations that had previously traded with each other in a market relationship vertically integrated and became a single organisation. Should a hospital run its own ambulance or pathology or A&E service or should it contract with a supplier of services? Will the costs of ensuring availability of a service of the reliability and quality desired be lower if provided internally, or if purchased from an independent organisation? The relevant costs are referred to as *transaction costs*. The relative size of these costs depends on the arrangements that must be put in place to monitor performance and adjust service requirements as, over time, unforeseen events require changes in service delivery that could not have been fully anticipated at the time a contract was negotiated.

In the analysis of these questions, NIE has added two additional concepts to those commonly used in economic analysis. *Bounded rationality* refers to the idea that there are important limits to the amount of information individuals can hold and process. Individuals are 'intendedly rational but only limitedly so' (Williamson 1986). *Opportunism* refers to the idea that as long as people have different objectives and information not possessed by others, they can be expected at times to behave in ways inconsistent with the objectives of the organisation or of their partners in a market exchange (Barney and Hesterly 1996). Under these conditions, the more specific the investments that one party has to make to satisfy the service requirements of the other, the more likely it is that transaction costs will be lower when organisations integrate. How transaction costs actually change with reconfiguration depends on a number of factors, including whether the cost of the risk of investments becoming redundant is reduced, and whether the costs of monitoring and providing incentives for good performance are lower within an organisation than between organisations. This is fundamentally an empirical issue (Croxson 1999).

To date the main application of the NIE framework to health services has focused on the economics of contracting (Dawson and Goddard 1999). A major problem has been how to measure the activities associated with the concept of transaction cost (Place *et al.*). While we are at the early stages of identifying the difference in costs and performance of organising services within a single organisation (e.g. general practitioners who own and run community hospitals) as opposed to organising services across organisations, the questions are high on the research agenda.

The analytical models of neo-classical economics and NIE are, in principle, as applicable to public-sector institutions as to private-sector institutions. Indeed part of the research agenda is to understand the factors that may lead organisations to perform more efficiently in one sector rather than the other. It is certainly the case that the volume of empirical research produced on private-sector health care services is significantly greater than that on public-sector health care services. However, this is a reflection of the fact that, historically, the public sector has collected and published much fewer data than, in some countries, regulators have required be produced by the private sector.

Uses

The research questions that can be investigated using the methods of economics are varied, but all linked to the management of scarcity. Figure 8.1 is a schematic presentation of the research agenda traditionally addressed by health economics.

Economic evaluation of interventions and organisation (Boxes E and G in Figure 8.1) is discussed in Chapter 7. Organisational economics ordinarily

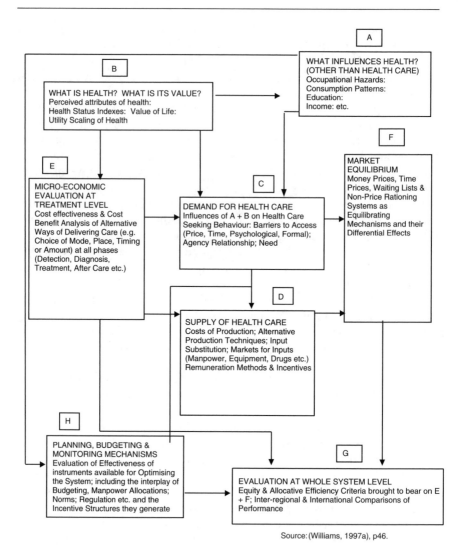

Figure 8.1 Structure of the discipline applied to health
Source: Williams 1997a: 46

focuses on the issues noted in Boxes C, D, F and H. Some examples are highlighted in the boxes of Figure 8.1; one example is described in more detail here.

Historically, an important set of research questions addressed by economists centred on the incentives generated by different methods of remuneration (Box D). Do clinicians paid on a fee-for-service basis prescribe more drugs, ask for more diagnostic tests, refer a higher proportion of patients for more surgical interventions than clinicians paid by capitation or salary? The answer has been a clear yes, with important implications for reform in the organisation of health services in a number of countries. Similar issues have been explored in research on methods for remunerating hospitals. All of these effects were predicted by economic theory but required empirical verification. Traditionally, clinicians argued that their decisions on what drugs to prescribe or whether to offer a patient coronary artery bypass surgery were determined purely by clinical need. The cumulative empirical research of several decades has demonstrated that this is not the case, and that the economic framework within which clinicians function makes an important difference to the treatments they provide to their patients.

Figure 8.2 provides a different perspective on the questions addressed by economic research, in this case with a focus on institutional elements. Theory predicts that the transaction costs of organising services will differ as between public and private sectors, profit and not-for-profit, market and non-market delivery. The arrows indicate possible combinations of institutional arrangements that may be the focus of research. For example, one may want to study differences in health service delivery of systems where hospitals are in the private sector (1), some are not-for-profit organisations (4) and some are for-profit organisations (3) but each must compete with other providers for income (5). This example would correspond to the dominant configuration in the USA. One might wish to examine the outcomes of an alternative institutional arrangement embracing public-sector providers (2) operating on a not-for-profit basis (4) but where they must compete with other providers for income (5). This was expected to be the model of the internal market in the National Health Service in the UK the 1990s. Typical research questions would be whether the alternative institutional arrangements affect selection of patients for treatment, costs of treatment or health outcomes.

In most health care systems, purchasers have a choice of providers and this increases the importance of market incentive structures. However, non-market delivery (6) remains an important alternative. Perhaps the quantitatively most important examples at present are research councils (public sector) and charities (private sector) that fund medical and health services research. A major debate on the role of market as compared to non-market organisation was stimulated by Titmuss' analysis of alternative ways of organising the collection of blood for distribution to hospitals (Titmuss 1997; Solow 1971; Arrow 1974).

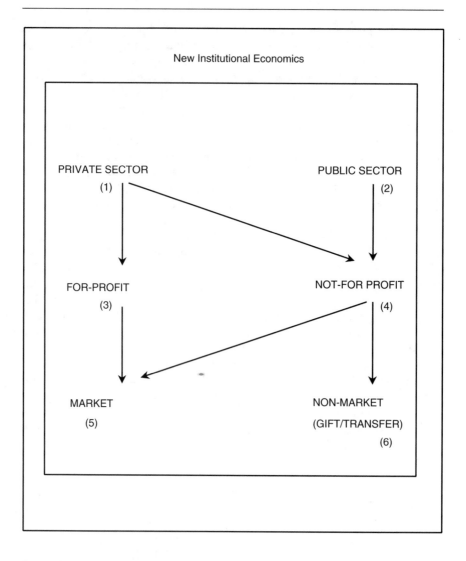

Figure 8.2 Elements in the economic modelling of health services organisation

How to undertake organisational economic research

Economics addresses a distinctive set of questions, employing a unique set of concepts, but the methods employed in empirical research are common to most social sciences. The principal methods are:

- econometrics (behavioural models plus statistics)

- qualitative analysis
- experimental

Looking at the published empirical research on health services, econometrics is the most frequently used method. There are several reasons for this dominance. First is the issue of 'generalisability'. Econometric studies use large data sets and allow for statistical generalisation. Econometric methods are also favoured because they offer the potential to test hypotheses on the population actually delivering or receiving a service, and not just those individuals included in highly controlled trials. In econometric models it is possible to control explicitly for factors expected to affect the relationships under examination – we do not have to assume teaching status affects quality of outcomes, we can test for the expected effect (see Box 8.1). In these models it is possible to study and quantify the interaction of variables

---

Box 8.1 Economic study of the impact of GP fundholding in the UK

With the development of a primary care-led NHS in the UK, an important issue is identification of effective incentive structures that will enable GPs to obtain improved services for their patients. During the 1990s there was a natural experiment where GP fundholders had some powers to influence provider behaviour for certain of their patients but not for others. Several case studies had suggested that fundholders were able to obtain improved service in terms of shorter waiting times for all their patients, and other studies suggested that patients of non-fundholding practices might be benefiting from the changes in provider behaviour stimulated by fundholders. The evidence was inconclusive and conflicting.

Propper and colleagues (Propper et al. 2000; Croxson et al. 1999) created a database from the CMDS that covered all elective admissions (138,800 admissions) from all GP practices in a health region over a period of four years. The results were clear. GPs were able to get shorter waiting times for those of their patients for whom they had the power to switch funding between providers. They did not appear to secure better waiting times for those of their patients for whom they lacked credible financial muscle, and patients of non-fundholding practices did not appear to benefit from changes in provider behaviour towards fundholders. There were important lessons for the development of incentive mechanisms for the NHS.

of key importance, such as the risk of no bed being available and the success of hospitals meeting cost performance targets (Bagust 1999). The statistical and modelling techniques used in econometric studies are similar to those discussed in respect of operational research (Chapter 10) and epidemiological research (Chapter 4).

A second reason for the prevalence of econometric techniques centres on cost and value for money. Econometric tests of ideas normally rely on the availability of routinely collected data. Ordinarily, if a new data set has to be collected, the costs will be very high. Few research studies (outside of privately funded clinical trials) can afford to collect such data. Not only is research using routinely collected data cheaper than having to generate data, it is also the data that governments and managers use to regulate health services. Research using these data is easier to transfer into policy. But there is a problem: remember Goodhart's Law, mentioned earlier? When an activity index is used for performance management, there is an incentive for hospitals to massage the coding of cases to improve apparent performance. Because policy makers use routine data in control mechanisms, researchers must be constantly aware of distortions that may consequently be introduced into the data.

The sources of data used in econometric studies differ by country. For the UK, currently the most important data set is the Contract Minimum Data Set (CMDS) that records data on each patient treated as an inpatient or day case in hospital. In addition to data on the patient – age, sex, method of admission (emergency, elective, etc.) diagnosis, procedure, place of discharge – it includes identifiers for the patient's primary care practice, hospital consultant, provider and purchaser. In recent years, data on health services have been made more useful by the availability of case-mix data. In most countries this is based on Diagnosis Related Group (DRG) classifications or some local variant, for example Healthcare Resource Groups (HRGs) in the UK. The other final important source of quantitative data is the set of Hospital Reference Costs, published on an annual basis. The data set out accounting costs by HRG for all acute hospitals. Given the title of this chapter, it is important to note that accounting costs do not correspond to economic costs, but at least these data provide the first opportunity in the UK to explore disaggregated hospital accounting costs at the level of individual procedures.

The major alternative to the quantitative analysis used in econometrics is qualitative analysis. There are several advantages of this technique. First, where theoretical models predict particular outcomes but relevant quantitative data do not exist, case studies may be the only way to identify the relevance of the predicted outcomes. Historically, quantitative data available on health services have been very poor, and case studies using qualitative data are one of the few means of improving our understanding of performance. This is especially true of public health care systems, where traditionally much fewer data are collected on service provision than in private health care systems (see Box 8.2). Perhaps the strongest argument for use of qualitative techniques is that they permit the refinement of hypotheses in the light of better knowledge of the institutional environment (Dugger 1994). In some cases, knowledge gained from case studies can also be used to refine and test models on a larger population. See Chapters 2 and 3 for further discussion of these methods.

Box 8.2 Qualitative study of the relative merits of different performance information

The NHS is attaching considerable policy importance to performance indicators and using quantitative information to single out good and bad performers. It is well known that there are statistical problems with league tables generated by performance indicators (Dawson and Street 2000; Gravelle et al. 2000), but it is also possible that non-quantifiable information (soft information) is more useful in judging performance than the hard information of quantifiable performance.

Goddard et al. (1999) used qualitative techniques to investigate the relative importance of hard and soft information in the evaluation of hospital performance. The research was based on case studies of eight hospitals located in two regions of England. Senior health service staff were asked to identify two hospitals which they considered were performing well, and two of the worst hospitals in their area. Semi-structured interviews were conducted with staff responsible for monitoring hospitals, with purchasers and with staff within the hospitals – forty semi-structured interviews in total. It was clear that in a number of cases soft information was considered more reliable than hard, that informal networks of communication were vital to monitoring performance and could be put in jeopardy by increasing use of hard performance indicators. There appeared to be important lessons for the way in which the new performance framework for the NHS should be developed.

Experimental methods are still rare in economics, but awareness of their methodological importance is growing (Hey 1991). Perhaps the best-known example in health economics is the RAND study, designed to identify the effects on utilisation, quality and costs of alternative ways of paying providers – fee-for-service, capitation or co-payment (Manning 1984) (see Box 8.3). Where the research question requires carefully controlled condi-

---

Box 8.3 The RAND health insurance experiment

The study randomly assigned people in six areas in the USA to different health insurance plans for periods of three or five years. Around 2,000 individuals under the age of sixty-five were included in the experiment. The aim of the study was to test the response of people to different charges for using health services in experimental conditions. Some people were enrolled in plans that provided care free at the point of use. Others had to pay varying proportions of the cost. For those paying some part of the cost there was usually a maximum annual payment. The study measured use of health services, health status, and the satisfaction of patients.

The study found that use of health services varied with the level of charges paid by patients directly. Those who faced large co-payments used services less. The reduction applied to most types of service from medication to hospitalisation. The exceptions were children's hospital services and some mental health services, which were not affected by the price at the point of access. In essence, health services were like other economic goods – their use was increased by low prices and decreased by higher ones.

Another aim of the study was to test for the response of providers of health care to different forms of payment, fee-for-service as opposed to capitation. While there was little difference for most services, rates of hospitalisation and length of stay were significantly lower in the capitated group. The form of payment did affect the behaviour of clinicians.

The study found that the effects of reduced use of health services on health were, at most, small. An important exception to this general finding was that the reduced use by poorer people did have a measurable and harmful effect on health.

(Newhouse 1993)

---

tions to test a hypothesis, a randomised study may provide more useful results than a non-randomised one. Where actual experimental methods are not possible, vignettes can be used to generate hypothetical alternatives (see Box 8.4).

Box 8.4 Why do GP referral rates differ? An experimental study

Variation in GP referral rates has long been recognised as a fact, and perceived as an important policy problem – there are implications for equity, hospital activity and waiting lists. The British NHS is seeking ways of reducing inappropriate variations. The problem is: what constitutes an inappropriate variation in the referrals by one GP relative to another? Econometric work can explain some of the variation, but observational studies cannot confront different GPs with the same patient in order to clearly separate differences in GP decisions from differences in the patients they see.

Earwicker and Whynes (1998) devised a study using vignettes to separate GP decision criteria from the patients they saw by, in effect, presenting each GP with identical patients. Questionnaires were mailed to all GPs in Nottingham, with case histories of eight hypothetical patients with medical problems familiar to most GPs and details of available options for managing them. The strongest of the hypotheses tested was that GPs operate on a consistent hierarchy or ranking of cases in terms of 'relative need for referral' but select different absolute cut-off points. The results supported this hypothesis, and in the light of the research results the potential role of referral protocols in reducing variation in referral rates was examined.

(Earwicker and Whynes 1998)

Limitations

The research questions of economics and the methods of analysis employed mean that research undertaken within this framework is particularly useful for some purposes but less relevant for others.

Economic analysis is designed to deal with situations where people have different objectives. It is assumed that the objective function of a physician will always be different from that of a hospital manager or a patient. Human beings are different in their interests and in what they value, as well as in the information they possess. Economics therefore emphasises the creation of incentives to try to reduce the divergence of action that would otherwise follow from differences in people's objectives. Other disciplines may study ways of changing how people think, altering their values and objectives. This may be possible, and there are economists working with researchers from other disciplines on topics such as changing the culture within organisations (Davies *et al.* 2000). Economists do not assume that preferences or technology are fixed, but recognise that over the long term preferences are moulded by institutions (Bowles 1998). Even more important, it has been recognised that within the health care sector, technical change and the introduction of new products is endogenous (i.e. determined by factors in the system, not independent of them) (Weisbrod 1991). However, the fact that preferences change does not mean that individuals will arrive at a common set of interests. Research into ways of changing the interests of individuals, so that their values and objectives are more similar, requires a framework different from that of economics. But, since trying to make clinicians think more along the lines of hospital managers will take some time and may never be achieved anyway, the system may still need the work of economists on incentives to reduce the adverse consequences of differences in objectives.

To non-economists, perhaps the most important limitation of economic research as an input into policy is the focus on the scarcity issue, with the implications of different policies examined in terms of impacts on efficiency and equity. For example, many research studies have indicated that there are diseconomies of scale in hospitals – after adjusting for case-mix, intensity and other factors, costs per patient treated are higher in the largest hospitals than in smaller hospitals (Ferguson *et al.* 1997). However, some governments are observed to systematically encourage and promote mergers of hospitals in apparent disregard of the long-standing economics research evidence. The obvious implication is that the objectives relevant to the political decisions are different from those studied by economists. Observers interested in understanding the pattern of merger activity will need to consult the work of policy analysts rather than economists.

Williams has suggested that it is the methodology of economics that creates friction at the interface of economics with politics (Williams 1995; 1997b). Economic analysis requires the *explicit* statement of objectives and constraints in sufficiently precise terms, at a minimum, to identify conceptually optimal solutions (normative) or quantitatively to predict outcomes (positive). Being explicit about objectives is anathema to most political systems. In health care the best current example may be the discussion of rationing. This had been a core topic of economic analysis for the last forty years (at least), but until recently was an unacceptable concept for public political discourse.

To economists, the most important limitation on the usefulness of empirical health services research to date is the poor quality of data on patient outcomes. The entire methodological apparatus of economics is designed to understand the relationship between outcomes (outputs) and use of scarce resources. Studies of whether outreach clinics based in primary care are more efficient than traditional outpatient clinics based in hospitals, depend on having information on whether patient outcomes are the same or different under these alternative ways of organising the delivery of services. In the past, economists have been justly criticised for using activity measures such as number of patients treated or number of tests administered or intermediate outcomes, such as changes in cholesterol levels, as indicators of output. These indications cannot shed light on the extent to which the investment in health care is generating improvements in health states, which, within economics, is the object of the exercise. Recent developments in a number of countries mean we can expect more information on outcomes of health care in future, and this should mean that much more relevant and useful economic research will be possible (see Chapter 7).

Further reading

Bryman, A. I. and Burgess, R. G. (1999) *Qualitative Research*, London: Sage.

Clay, S. (1992) *Long-Term Contracting: A Bibliography and Review of the Literature*, Oxford: Centre for Socio-Legal Studies, Wolfson College.

Folland, S., Goodman, A. C. and Stano, M. (1997) *The Economics of Health and Health Care*, 2nd edn, New Jersey: Prentice-Hall.

Furubotn, E. G. and Richter, R. (2000) *Institutions and Economic Theory: The Contribution of the New Institutional Economics*, Ann Arbor: University of Michigan Press.

Jones, A. M. (2000) 'Health econometrics', in A. J. Culyer and J. P. Newhouse (eds) *Handbook of Health Economics*, Amsterdam: North Holland.

Kennedy, P. (1998) *A Guide to Econometrics*, Oxford: Blackwell.

McCloskey, D. N. (1985) *The Applied theory of Price*, 2nd edn, London: Collier-Macmillan.

Williamson, O. E. and Masten, S. E. (1995) *Transaction Cost Economics*, vols I and II, Aldershot: Edward Elgar.

References

Arrow, K. J. (1963) 'Uncertainty and the welfare economics of medical care', *The American Economic Review*, LIII: 941–73.

——(1974) 'Gifts and exchanges', *Philosophy and Public Affairs*, 1: 343–62.

Bagust, A. (1999) 'Dynamics of bed use in accommodating emergency admissions: stochastic simulation model', *British Medical Journal*, 319: 155–8.

Barney, J. B. and Hesterly, W. (1996) 'Organizational economics: understanding the relationship between organizations and economic analysis', in S. Clegg, C. Hardy and W. Nord (eds) *Handbook of Organizational Studies*, London: Sage.

Bowles, S. (1998) 'Endogenous preferences: the cultural consequences of markets and other economic institutions', *Journal of Economic Literature*, XXXVI: 75–111.

Caldwell, B. J. (1982) *Beyond Positivism: Economic Methodology in the Twentieth Century*, London: George Allen and Unwin.

Coast, J. (1999) 'The appropriate uses of qualitative methods in health economics', *Health Economics*, 8: 345–53.

Croxson, B. (1999) *Organisational Costs in the New NHS*, London: Office of Health Economics.

Croxson, B., Propper, C. and Perkins, A. (1999) 'Do doctors respond to financial incentives? UK family doctors and the GP fundholder scheme', *Journal of Public Economics*, 79: 375–98.

Culyer, A. J. and Newhouse, J. P. (2000) *Handbook of Health Economics*, Amsterdam: North Holland.

Davies, H. T. O., Nutley, S. M., Mannion, R. and Small, N. (2000) 'Organisational culture and quality of health care', *Quality in Health Care*, 9: 111–19.

Dawson, D. and Goddard, M. (1999) 'Long-term contracts in the NHS: a solution in search of a problem?', *Health Economics*, 8: 709–20.

Dawson, D. and Street, A. (2000) 'Comparing NHS hospital unit costs', *Public Money and Management*, 20, 4: 58–62.

Dugger, W. (1994) 'Methodological differences between institutional and neoclassical economics', in D. M. Hausman (ed.) *The Philosophy of Economics*, 336–44, Cambridge: Cambridge University Press.

Earwicker, S. C. and Whynes, D. K. (1998) 'General practitioners' referral thresholds and choices of referral destination: an experimental study', *Health Economics*, 7: 711–22.

Ferguson, B., Posnett, J. and Sheldon, T. (1997) *Concentration and Choice in the Provision of Hospital Services*, York: NHS Centre for Reviews and Dissemination.

Goddard, M., Mannion, R. and Smith, P. C. (1999) 'Assessing the performance of NHS hospital trusts: the role of "hard" and "soft" information', *Health Policy*, 48, 119–34.

Goodhart, C. A. E. (1984) *Monetary Theory and Practice: The UK experience*, London: Macmillan.

Gravelle, H., Dusheiko, M. and Sutton, M. (2000) 'Rationing by time, distance and money in the NHS: variations in admission rates', Technical Paper Series no. TP17, York: Centre for Health Economics.

Hey, J. D. (1991) *Experiments in Economics*, Oxford: Blackwell.

Manning, W. G. (1984) 'A controlled trial of the effect of a pre-paid group practice on use of services', *New England Journal of Medicine*, 310: 1505–10.

Mannion, R. and Small, N. (1999) 'Postmodern health economics', *Health Care Analysis*, 7: 255–72.

Newhouse, J. P. (1993) *Free for All: Lessons from the RAND Health Insurance Experiment*, Cambridge MA: Harvard University Press.

Place, M., Posnett, J. and Street, A. (1998) *An Analysis of the Transactions Costs of Total Purchasing Pilots*, London: King's Fund.

Propper, C., Croxson, B. and Shearer, A. (2000) *Waiting Times for Hospital Admissions: The Impact of GP Fundholding*, Discussion Paper 00/20, Bristol: Centre for Market and Public Organisation.

Robbins, L. (1984) *An Essay on the Nature and Significance of Economic Science*, London: Macmillan.

Solow, R. M. (1971) 'Blood and thunder (review)', *Yale Law Journal*, 80: 1696–711.

——(1997) 'How did economics get that way and what way did it get?', *Daedalus*, 126: 39–58.

Titmuss, R. M. (1997) *The Gift Relationship*, London: LSE Books.

Weisbrod, B. (1991) 'The health care quadrilemma: an essay on technological change, insurance, quality of care and cost containment', *Journal of Economic Literature*, XXIX: 523–52.

Williams, A. (1995) 'The role of quantitative modelling in health care', *Health Economics*, 4: 1–6.

——(1997a) 'Health economics: the cheerful face of the dismal science?', in A. J. Culyer and A. Maynard (eds) *Being Reasonable about the Economics of Health*, 45–53, Cheltenham: Edward Elgar.

——(1997b) 'Cost-benefit analysis: bastard science and/or insidious poison in the body politick?', in A. J. Culyer and A. Maynard (eds) *Being Reasonable about the Economics of Health*, 3–25, Cheltenham: Edward Elgar.

Williamson, O. E. (1986) 'What is transaction cost economics?', in *Economic Organization*, 174–96, Brighton: Wheatsheaf Books.

Chapter 9

Historical research

Virginia Berridge

Introduction

This chapter looks at historical methods, their theoretical bases and uses, and gives some idea of how historians construct their accounts and the sources they use. In common parlance, history is just 'one damn thing after another'. But historical research is an intensely theoretical activity, a dimension often ignored by those who assume historians are simply 'fact gatherers'. The types of historical method used and the 'facts' selected as relevant are all determined by a historian's theoretical position. Analyses and interpretations are themselves socially and historically located.

Definition and theoretical basis

The dominant historiographical tendencies also have implications for methodology and for analysis. The major trends in historical writing about health and health services over the past thirty to forty years have seen a move away from notions of historical progress, where the past was seen as a precursor to the achievements of the present. This style of historical writing is known as 'Whig history' after the eighteenth-century British political party which represented a progressive view of history.

For medicine, this was the 'old doctors'' view of history, which necessarily privileged the breakthroughs and discoveries of the present. It tended to downplay lay perspectives and the views of non-medical workers, and assumed that certain tendencies had 'won' because they were 'right'. The losers in history lost because they deserved to.

The 1960s, which saw an emergent critical response to the role of medicine in society more generally, provoked a critique of Whig history, aided by an influx of non-medical historians into the field as part of a more general expansion of social history. Different types of history emerged, and research began to look at the nature of the family, the role of women and children, the social construction of disease categories and lay perspectives (Webster 1993). Sociological theories were drawn upon in order to analyse the social and cultural dimensions of science and medicine. Foucault was first discovered by historians, and his insights used extensively in work on madness and deviance (Jones and Porter 1994). Anthropological work was used in the discussion of culture and of the boundaries between religion, medicine and magic. More recently, other theoretical inputs have assumed prominence, with interest in the body, consumption and commodification, representation and discourse, literary theory and identity. The postmodern critique of the entire historical enterprise has occasioned much debate, and has implications for methods and for analysis which will be discussed below (Munslow 1999).

To understand the interrelationships between science and policy, two theoretical schools can be drawn on. One is policy science, with its interest in the nature of policymaking, power within society, and the role of networks within the policy process (see Chapter 6) (Marsh and Rhodes 1992). The other is a development of social constructionism – the sociology of scientific knowledge, with its interest derived from Latour in 'actor networks' in the production of science (Latour 1987). However, Rodney Lowe argues that while it is advisable to be theoretically informed, it is not advisable to spend huge amounts of time on theoretical development (Lowe 1999). That leads to less time for the sources, which have to be the bedrock of historical analysis. 'Real historians' immerse themselves in their primary sources with a theoretical perspective in mind, rather than plunging into those sources in order to validate theory.

That brings us back to the idea of 'facts' in history. E. H. Carr, in his famous *What Is History?*, said that there was no such thing as a fact until it was created by historians (Carr 1986). More recently, Richard Evans has argued rather that 'facts' are there but that theory and interpretation come in when facts are converted into evidence (Evans 1997). History can be theoretically eclectic, which is seen is atheoreticism by those outside the discipline. Historical writing can also be monotheoretical, using a particular brand of theory to inform the primary source material.

Uses of historical research

History is unusual in two ways: in asking big questions and in dealing with change. It might not answer the 'what works?' type of question, but it might, for example, throw light on:

- Why and how do we have our current health systems? How and why do they differ from the past?
- What have been the key factors, persons, institutions, professions, social mechanisms, cultures which have given us the systems we have now?
- What alternative models are possible and how have they operated in the past?

- What has been the interrelationship between voluntary and statutory systems over time? Why and how has this changed? How have boundaries worked in the past? What has been the history of the relationship between hospitals and primary health care? Why do hospitals resist amalgamation? How have their histories differed?
- How have lay and professional boundaries changed and why?
- How and why have systems differed between countries?
- Are our preconceptions about the way services work, have impact and develop supported by historical evidence and the nature of change over time?
- How and for what reasons have different health professions established their areas of competence, and how have boundaries been established?
- Why are health services problems defined as they are?

These types of question can be honed down into more specific areas dependent on the topic under consideration (see Boxes 9.1 and 9.2).

Box 9.1 The way a health system has developed

Charles Webster's official history of the National Health Service in the UK, and accounts written by others, have shown the broad way services developed (Webster 1988; 1996). Webster has criticised the notion of consensus posited by Klein (1995) and others about the formation of the NHS (Webster 1990). This interpretation has been carried forward by Harriet Jones' work on the role of consensus and the post-war Conservative government, where she shows that the Conservatives would have liked to reduce the welfare state but were prevented by electoral considerations (Jones 1991). Lowe has argued that the formation of the NHS, far from being a triumph, was a gigantic missed opportunity which has dogged its operation ever since (Lowe 1999). There has also been much recent work on the inter-war health services, previously condemned as a complex and ineffective patchwork. The apparent revival of some of the organisational complexity of the 1930s in the 1980s has led to comparisons between the two periods. A paper by Martin Powell compared health services in the 1980s and 1990s with those of the 1930s, and found that there was much similarity (Powell 1996). The absence of democracy in the NHS was the major difference between the two periods. Health services in the inter-war period had more democratic control, and this 'democratic deficit' has been a major feature of the operation of the NHS.

> **Box 9.2 How specialities have developed**
>
> For public health and primary care in the UK, Jane Lewis' work on community medicine and its relationship to social medicine, and later to the developing concept of primary health care, has been important. She has developed a critique of public health and its ideology (or lack of it) and also pointed to the continuing tensions, both pre- and post-war, between general practitioners and public health doctors for the same terrain (Lewis 1986). Other historical work has looked at the origins of divisions, which we now take for granted, between general practitioners and hospital consultants, or at the post-war history of the way in which general practice developed.
>
> (Loudon et al. 1998)

Historians would be wary about drawing direct 'lessons' from historical analyses. Instead, they widen the debate, not least in giving validity to different perspectives on the present. This is a classic historical function – of making what seems obvious and self-evident in the present problematic and strange.

How to undertake historical research

Data sources

Historians, whatever their theoretical stance, use a variety of sources. A key source is the existing work of other historians, so-called secondary sources. That is what is surveyed in this chapter's opening paragraph about trends in previous historical writing: it is called the historiography of the area.

The materials that historians find and use in their own work are known as primary sources. These are the evidence on which they base their interpretations. For the sake of clarity, three types of primary source can be identified: documentary, quantitative and oral. In practice, historians often use a combination of different forms of source material. Some of these sources overlap with those used by other disciplines, although the nature of the use is not always the same and the questions asked are different. For example, interviewing is used by many disciplines.

Documentary sources

Let's look first at documentary sources and imagine what they might consist of. Imagine you are transported to year 2100 and are researching some aspect of service development and organisation in 2000. What primary sources are being created in documentary form which you might call on a hundred years hence?

You might use some of the following: a mass media article or programme about the state of the health system; an official record of parliamentary debates; a statistical survey; or the text of a government bill. There might be a transcript of interviews with politicians or civil servants deposited in an oral history archive. You would be able to access the minutes of meetings of a committee, and see the memoranda which had gone back and forth between civil servants, probably in their electronic form as well. The Minister of Health of the day or the leading politicians or civil servants (if permitted) might have written memoirs after they retired.

This is by no means an exhaustive list but it gives an indication. One of the problems of historical research is the overabundance of materials for the more recent period. Some primary sources are easy to access, for example, newspapers, which are now often available in CD-ROM as well as paper or microfilm copies. Others are more difficult, involving negotiation over access to diaries or letters or requests for access to more recent governmental material. For more recent history, historians have to seek out their own sources. Close relationships with 'living historical actors' often lead to archival finds, and historians can end up partly acting as archivists as well. I was recently introduced at a doctors' conference as an 'avid archivist', which is not quite what I am, but it gave the right impression to the medical and scientific audience who might have potential data to offer.

Quantitative sources

There are many ways of using quantitative sources in historical work. There are published statistics of mortality over time, and these are used graphically in published accounts of the health of the public. When I was writing a survey book on post-war health and society in Britain, I searched out statistics on hospital bed occupancy, on numbers of beds available and how that had changed over time (Berridge 1999).

Statistical sources can also be created or moulded from other quantitative raw material. Hospital yearbooks have been much used by British historians looking at the operation of health services between the World Wars (Cherry 1996). Other research has used published annual statistics to look at bed occupancy rates and to contribute to an argument about the validity of the costings that formed part of discussions at the inception of the NHS in Britain (Cutler 2000). Patient records have been used also in quantitative, computer-based form. Mental health records have shown the patterns of patients' movement in and out of asylums, and have contributed to historical debates, with contemporary resonance, about the function of the asylum.

There are advantages to the use of this type of data – the ability to discern patterns over time, to assess perceptions against reality, and to arrive at a more precise estimation of change. But there are also disadvantages. Statistical tables and their construction are not value-free, and the way in which they are compiled may change. But non-historians are more comfortable with them, as they seem to offer a form of certainty, however spurious, which parallels data used in other scientific analysis.

Oral history

Much experience is neither quantified nor written down. Oral accounts can be revealing. Usually these are gathered from individuals through interviewing. Oral history has come to prominence as a historical method in the last thirty or so years, in connection initially with newer inputs into historical work, in particular labour, social and feminist history. Mainstream Whig history tended to focus only on the study of 'great events' and 'great men' (rarely women), accepting the perspective of the dominant forces and perspectives in society – the history of the winners. From the 1960s onward, there were moves to challenge these views of the past and to write history from the perspective of those who had left few written records. This was 'history from below'.

This was associated in Britain with the Oral History Society, Paul Thompson's work and the History Workshop movement. The main advantage was that it could reveal aspects of social history which were not written down, such as the patient's perspective or work practices. It was especially important for women's history, which does not emerge from the documentary sources (Thompson and Perks 1993).

Methods of doing oral history have varied – some have used a quota survey, others take a snowball sample. For example, a study based on oral histories of community pharmacists in the UK interviewed some of those who qualified in each decade, who practised in different geographical areas, and who came from different ethnic backgrounds (Anderson and Berridge 1999). Michael Bevan's oral histories of general practice covered the whole country (Bevan 1999). Another similar study is located in Paisley, Scotland, covering that one town to analyse the local and particular context. Oral history may be combined with documentary and other sources (see Box 9.2).

Oral history is also a tool to record the experience of elites in society. Sometimes historians use the equivalent of a 'focus group' for elite oral history – the 'witness seminar'. For example, a 'witness seminar' on the Black Report (a report commissioned by the British government) on health inequalities in the UK, which was published in 1980, produced new insights into why the Report achieved such notoriety (Berridge and Blume [in press]). Witness seminars are a valuable tool for recent history, especially where documents are not available.

The disadvantages of oral history can be summarised as memories of a 'golden age', settling old scores, and the danger that people, especially eminent ones, will be over-interviewed. There has been much discussion in the oral history field recently on the nature of memory and of different views of time as displayed in oral testimony. Its relationship to the documentary sources can be complex. In researching the history of UK AIDS policy, one key oral history source subsequently provided access to the papers of a committee on which he had served (Box 9.3). Those papers were invaluable, not because they undermined his oral testimony, but because they complemented and expanded on it, in particular in raising issues which otherwise would have gone undiscussed (Berridge 1996).

Box 9.3 Understanding how health care policy develops

Recently, historians have begun to work on quite recent health history. Work on AIDS policy making in the UK in the 1980s and early 1990s used oral interviews with clinicians, gay men, scientists and others, as well as archival material, to look at the interplay between 'bottom-up' and 'top-down' policy making, at the extraordinary crisis period of 1986–7, and at the nature of the liberal consensus formed during a period of ostensible right-wing reaction in government. Historical work has here sought to counter easy interpretations which talk of 'moral panic' or of 'delay' in reactions, or which look back with hindsight – always a problem with writing about more recent history (Berridge 1996).

Rafferty's (1996) work on the history of the development of nurse education in the UK from the 1860s to the 1940s highlights the influence of policy models outside the health sector, particularly from the education sector. The model of organisation for nurse education in the early twentieth century was heavily influenced by organisational models developed by the Department of Education. Rafferty notes that these 'policy seepages' are often influenced by the movement of civil servants between government departments. Parallels can be seen today in the development of the Commission for Health Improvement, established in 1999 to improve standards of care in the NHS, based at least in part on the concept of the Office for Standards in Education (Ofsted) set up in 1992.

Data collection methods

There is a difference between ideal and actual, certainly in terms of starting research. There are some good guides to how to get started, and there has been a great expansion of aids to finding material in recent years. The website of the University of London's Institute of Historical Research has links to many of these (http://www.ihrinfo.ac.uk). There is Histline and the Wellcome online library catalogue which can be searched by subject (http://www.wellcome.ac.uk).

The danger is an overabundance of material from which to start. Work on the policy history of nicotine replacement therapy turned up over 400 items from an initial bibliographic search. Secondary material is where to start, with a few references of good quality garnered through initial reading, or recommended by colleagues. Further work can then be built on those references and an initial plan of primary source research developed. For initial primary research, dependent on topic, searches through key health care journals are a helpful starting point in order to develop an initial sense of the shape of the issue and its development over time. This is where starting historical research differs from other ways of reviewing literature (see Chapter 12). There the emphasis is often on electronic databases, which cover quite short periods of past time and omit particular forms or ranges of publication (books and most historical journals, for example).

Modes of analysis

Broad theoretical positioning, referred to earlier, does not mean that historians start out with a hypothesis they are testing. The approach is deductive, a form of interaction with the source material in order to develop an interpretation. Not all the evidence can be used – or even researched in the first place – so historians have to be careful that they are weighing up different types of evidence, and make sure they are not constructing an analysis which simply confirms their own preconceptions. Research and analysis is a matter of constant reassessment and revision in the light of the sources. It is not just a question of 'uncovering the facts' as some kind of academic detective story, but of discovering and examining evidence and then of compiling evidence in a coherent form (Box 9.4). As Mary James says, 'using experience and imagination to construct these into a meaningful account' (James 1994). The resultant text is an interpretation, not 'the facts'.

Box 9.4 Kidney dialysis – understanding why and how covert rationing takes place

Kidney dialysis has often been cited – from Aaron and Schwartz in the 1970s to Rudolf Klein on the NHS in the 1990s (Stanton 1999) – as a prime example of covert or implicit rationing in the British NHS, obvious enough when UK figures on provision of dialysis compared so unfavourably with those of other European countries (and were about half those in the USA in the 1970s). However, to understand why it persisted and how it operated requires historical methods. Through interviews, reading the contemporary medical literature of the 1960s to 1980s with an eye to themes of patient selection, plus looking at papers of governmental advisory groups, parliament, and accounts by patients and patient support groups, notable themes emerge, often with relevance for the present day (Stanton 1999):

- The role of the general practitioner or non-specialist hospital physician in acting as a 'gatekeeper' so as to limit referrals for dialysis was not surprising (such a role is evident in many other cases), but how were the parameters set? They seem to have been laid down in the pioneer period when renal physicians wanting to prove the benefits of the treatment to sceptical funders chose the most suitable patients – i.e. those fit enough to survive. Gradually more categories were added, but the idea persisted that the elderly were less likely to benefit. The use of language around this issue has been very revealing.
- Voluntary group campaigning did help to put dialysis on the policy agenda, but failed to achieve its main aim (revealed in parliamentary questions), namely to change UK laws to ensure everyone's organs were donated on death unless they opted out. Most politicians viewed this as a move the British population was not ready to contemplate.
- By tracing the relation of other social science disciplines to health, historical methods reveal that even the most sought-after inputs – such as the tools of health economics – had little impact when the question of rationing dialysis was gaining publicity. Quantitative measures of survival and quality of life were demonstrating the relatively poor cost-benefit of dialysis just when the government decided to impose targets to increase dialysis provision in 1984. On the other hand, a health economics approach that suited the ideology of the government of the day – the internal market – was adopted, and dialysis was an arena for early experiments in encouraging the private sector to invest capital in the NHS.
- Crude comparisons between units, regions and countries have tended to carry more policy valency than most other types of research, possibly because of their media impact.

Recent postmodern debates about history have cast doubt on this way of doing history. Postmodernists argue that historical texts are 'heavily authored second hand knowledge constituted and organised by the historian' (Munslow 1999). Postmodern critics of the historical enterprise argue that historians must turn away from the belief that they can recover the meaning of the past, and argue for a history that is determined by moral and non-empiricist positions. Some historians like Evans (1997) have responded robustly to these criticisms, as they represent issues of which they have long been aware.

At a basic level, analysis is carried out through the interrogation of each source for meaning – trying to understand the intent of the source and the context in which it was produced. There is no such thing as an unbiased source – the biases of the particular source have to be understood. A source needs to be assessed in the context of its own time rather than imposing later categories on it.

Evidence is then interwoven into an analytic frame – this is the process which is called triangulation by other disciplines (see Chapter 1) (Silverman 1993). But historians, in general, are not so explicit about methodological discussion. The validity of the process is supported rather through footnotes, peer assessment and experience. I noticed, travelling home from a conference with another historian when we had books to review, that we both turned first to the end of our books and studied the bibliographies and the footnotes. We needed to know what primary source and what secondary material the authors had used, in order to make an initial assessment of the likely validity of the conclusions. Historians might argue that other disciplines have theorised and standardised these processes of analysis in an attempt to prove that they are scientific. Being scientific has not worried historians so much, although some earlier historians did mimic the scientific method in the 'history laboratory' (Birch and Horn 1996).

So how do historians establish validity, in the scientific sense? Does more than one historian work on the same sets of primary data to see if they came up with the same conclusions? This question brings home the gulf between different systems of analysis. Using primary sources is not a predetermined process; two historians starting from the same initial point would need to find their own ways through the primary data. That might lead to different pathways, both in terms of the material used and considered significant, and in terms of the ultimate analysis. Even if the same material were used, different or complementary conclusions might be reached. But those analyses, however different, would advance understanding.

Four recent books on the history of the international drug trade and drug control which had used much source material in common had each developed very different analyses and emphases (Berridge 2001). This process of advancing understanding through historical research is at first sight different to the scientific mode. But it is no less valid. It is a process of accretion, of modification and revision of accepted positions, rather than the model of unified 'discovery' which animates science. Of course, sociologists and historians of science have shown that in reality the scientific method is not like that at all. It is much more akin to the historical model. And the contemporary perception of 'scientific method' as value-free is itself a historical construct. So in historical research, the processes are founded on individual interaction with the material, on apprenticeship, experience and peer assessment.

Limitations

The limitations of these methods may be clear. Above all, they deal with big issues and do not provide specific answers. However, they open up the issues and provide a wider forum for debate. Potentially they can change the framework within which issues are discussed.

Other limitations derive from two directions – the nature of health services research; and the nature of historical research, of historians and their culture.

Let us look at the nature of health services research first. Here it is apparent that historical work is not seen as a natural component. Historical research is rarely funded from health services research funds. This may, in part, be for structural and historical reasons. Historians have not been part of health services research in the way sociologists and health policy specialists have. But it is also because historians' mode of analysis is difficult to handle. It can be too challenging or too wide-ranging, opening up issues that are not really in the immediate frame. The image of what history is can cause it to be discounted. If potential users think history is 'the facts', then anyone can use them. We all know those texts which throw in a few hastily assembled dates and events as justification for present-day concerns. On the other hand, if history is conceptual on a large scale it does not provide direct answers but only makes things more complicated.

Then there is the nature of historical research, of historians and their culture. There are a number of potential difficulties here, not least practical ones. Historians, however eminent, cannot give up direct hands-on research. The highest level of expertise is needed to interact with the primary source material. This is not an exercise which is easily delegated to less experienced research fellows, or to a team (as with micro-level qualitative research discussed in Chapter 3). Historians therefore operate in different ways from the great body of health services researchers, and often over longer timescales. A typical primary research grant would be two or three years in length, though shorter timescales are possible. Historical literature reviews can be commissioned to be completed over much shorter periods of time, and can help to inform agendas.

Many historians are unaware of the significance of what they are studying in present-day terms. There is even some resistance to being 'policy relevant'. Not many historians work in health services research settings where they can develop awareness of contemporary policy issues. Few are members of expert committees in their capacity as historians. When I worked in a policy-relevant post for a while, I had to drop any idea of being overtly an historian. My committee did not want to be reminded that some of their concerns had historical roots. More recently I have given 'expert' evidence to an official committee which did have a substantial historical component in its final report and a historian as its research worker. But the implications of the historical material were not developed in the report's conclusions, and the members of the committee grew increasingly uneasy about taking them on board in a controversial area. The interpretive culture of history also means that few historians will put themselves 'on the line' about the way in which policy should go. While the postmodern school argues that history should be partisan, the dominant historical stance is still what Evans calls a detached mode of cognition, which one should adopt even if there is a moral or political purpose to writing.

Historical research can influence policy makers, as the example of policy making on HIV and AIDS in the 1980s demonstrates. In an area where there was no policy template to guide action, politicians did turn directly to historical analogy (Berridge 1996). Historical arguments for a non-punitive response were of key importance. In less dramatic instances, historical arguments have informed and challenged contemporary preconceptions. One example is the continuing debate in Britain about the location of control of health services and the role of local government, which was fatally weakened by the establishment of the NHS in 1948. However, politicians can choose to ignore history, as they seem to be doing in current moves to relocate parts of social services from local government to the NHS, with its predominant medical model. History's different, but no less valid, methodological and conceptual approaches should not undermine the value of history for health services research. From another perspective these are strengths. History is the key to the 'big picture' and to the overall dynamic and questioning analysis that is so often lacking in health policy discussions.

Further reading

Berridge, V. (1999) *Health and Society in Britain since 1939*, Cambridge: Cambridge University Press.

Carr, E. H. (1986) *What is History?*, Basingstoke: Macmillan.

Evans, R. J. (1997) *In Defence of History*, London: Granta.

Institute of Historical Research website, University of London, http://www.ihrinfo.ac.uk

James, M. (1994) 'Historical research methods', in K. McConway (ed.) *Studying Health and Disease*, Milton Keynes: Open University Press.

Lewis, J. (1986) *What Price Community Medicine? The Philosophy, Practice and Politics of Public Health since 1919*, Brighton: Harvester/Wheatsheaf.

Lowe, R. (1999) *The Welfare State in Britain since 1945*, 2nd edn, Basingstoke: Macmillan.

Thompson, P. and Perks, R. (1993) *An Introduction to the Use of Oral History in the History of Medicine*, London: British Sound Archive.

Webster, C. (ed.) (1993) *Caring for Health: History and Diversity*, Milton Keynes: Open University Press.

Wellcome website, http://www.wellcome.ac.uk

References

Anderson, S. and Berridge, V. (1999) 'The role of the community pharmacist in health and welfare 1911–1986', in J. Bornat, R. Perks, P. Thompson, and J. Walmsley (eds) *Oral History, Health and Welfare*, London: Routledge.

Berridge, V. (1996) *AIDS in the UK: The Making of Policy, 1981–1994*, Oxford: Oxford University Press.

——(1999) *Health and Society in Britain since 1939*, Cambridge: Cambridge University Press.

——(2001) 'Illicit drugs and internationalism: the forgotten dimension', *Medical History*, forthcoming.

Berridge, V. and Blume, S. (eds) (in press) *Contemporary British History*, special issue on 'Inequalities in health'.

Bevan, M. (1999) 'Family and vocation: career choice and the life histories of general practitioners', in J. Bornat, R. Perks, P. Thompson and J. Walmsley (eds) *Oral History, Health and Welfare*, London: Routledge.

Birch, D. and Horn, J. (1996) *The History Laboratory: The Institute of Historical Research 1921–1996*, London: Institute of Historical Research.

Carr, E. H. (1986) *What is History?*, Basingstoke: Macmillan.

Cherry, S. (1996) *Medical Services and the Hospitals in Britain, 1860–1939*, Cambridge: Cambridge University Press.

Cutler, T. (2000) 'The cost of the National Health Service: problem definition and policy response, 1942–1960', Ph.D. thesis, London School of Hygiene and Tropical Medicine, University of London.

Evans, R. J. (1997) *In Defence of History*, London: Granta.

James, M. (1994) 'Historical research methods', in K. McConway (ed.) *Studying Health and Disease*, Milton Keynes: Open University Press.

Jones, C. and Porter, R. (1994) *Reassessing Foucault: Power, Medicine and the Body*, London: Routledge.

Jones, H. (1991) 'New tricks for an old dog? The Conservatives and social policy, 1951–1955', in A. Gorst, L. Johnman and W. Scott-Lucas (eds) *Contemporary British History, 1931–1961: Politics and the Limits of Policy*, London: Pinter.

Klein, R. (1995) *The New Politics of the NHS*, 3rd edn, London: Longman.

Latour, B. (1987) *Science in Action: How to Follow Scientists and Engineers through Society*, Milton Keynes: Open University Press.

Lewis, J. (1986) *What Price Community Medicine? The Philosophy, Practice and Politics of Public Health since 1919*, Brighton: Harvester/Wheatsheaf.

Loudon, I., Horder, J. and Webster, C. (1998) *General Practice under the National Health Service, 1948–1997*, Oxford: Clarendon Press.

Lowe, R. (1999) *The Welfare State in Britain since 1945*, 2nd edn, Basingstoke: Macmillan.

Marsh, D. and Rhodes, R. A. W. (eds) (1992) *Policy Networks in British Government*, Oxford: Clarendon Press.

Munslow, A. (1999) 'The postmodern in history: a response to Professor O'Brien', *Institute of Historical Research Reviews in History*, available at http://www.ihrinfo.ac.uk

Powell, M. (1996) 'The ghost of health services past: comparing British health policy of the 1930s with the 1980s and the 1990s', *International Journal of Health Services*, 26, 2: 253–68.

Rafferty, A. M. (1996) *The Politics of Nursing Knowledge*, London: Routledge.

Silverman, D. (1993) *Interpreting Qualitative Data*, London: Sage.

Stanton, J. (1999) 'The cost of living: kidney dialysis, rationing and health economics in Britain, 1965–1996', *Social Science and Medicine*, 49: 1169–82.

Thompson, P. and Perks, R. (1993) *An Introduction to the Use of Oral History in the History of Medicine*, London: British Sound Archive.

Webster, C. (1988) *The Health Services since the War: I. Problems of Health Care – The National Health Service since 1957*, London: HMSO.

——(1990) 'Conflict and consensus: explaining the British health service', *Twentieth Century British History*, 1, 115–51.

——(1996) *The Health Services since the War: II. Government and Health Care – The British National Health Service, 1958–1979*, London: The Stationery Office.

Webster, C. (ed.) (1993) *Caring for Health: History and Diversity*, Milton Keynes: Open University Press.

Chapter 10

Operational research

Jonathan Rosenhead

Introduction

Operational research (OR) has research in its title. Its alternative name is 'management science'. But research is certainly not all that it does, and its version of science is certainly not of the laboratory variety. It is arguable that OR constitutes one of the key elements which will enable health service managers to respond to some of the pressing current issues of health service organisation and delivery. The move from evidence-based medicine to evidence-based policy; the rhetoric (at least) of 'joined-up government'; the refrain of 'whole-systems thinking' – all these play to the strengths of operational research.

Some of this can already be seen in practice. Recent UK government OR work has included the sizing and scoping for NHS Direct (a first-contact telephone or e-mail access system to the NHS), and capacity estimation for walk-in centres. This is classical OR of the best kind, employed on novel problem situations at the start of the twenty-first century. The potential is wider still.

Definition and theoretical basis

There is no established definition of OR. However, 'modelling' is generally regarded as the defining characteristic of OR. A plausible definition of the subject is:

> A process of offering aid to organisational decision making through the construction of a model representing the interaction of relevant factors, which can be used to clarify the implications of choice.

Some points of emphasis in this definition should be highlighted. First, OR is a *process*, involving interaction between analysts and those charged with the responsibility for decisions. Second, the model is not restricted to using objective measurements, but may use subjective or qualitative inputs. Third, the function of the analytic activity is not the scientific determination of some optimum, but the clarification of the consequences of alternative actions.

These emphases are relevant, given the trajectory of OR. It had its origins in World War II in the work of natural scientists working in the field on the improvement of military operations. (This account concentrates on UK experience, although there are national differences.) OR was taken up first by industry, then from the 1960s by government and public agencies, and more recently in retailing, finance and telecommunications. Operational researchers were frequently the first computer users in their organisations, and the activity became associated with a group of computerised techniques which are now seen as the classical tools of OR. Broadly, they claimed to 'solve' the problems they were used on. However, typically they demanded large quantities of high-quality data and so were safely applicable only to the sort of repetitive, tactical operations that would generate them. Figure 10.1 shows some of the current research tools and methods used by operational researchers, classified into 'classical', 'intermediate' and 'new wave'.

Linear programming is the most highly developed of the classical tools of operational research. There are many variants and specialised applications. Broadly, it finds the allocation, subject to constraints, of a number of scarce resources between competing uses, which maximises some performance measure. The underlying assumption is that both the performance function and the resource consumption are linearly related to the allocations.

The other main classical tool of OR is simulation, which is especially applicable where a system of interest consists of a number of interacting activities whose durations are probabilistic. A computer model of the interactions and probability distributions of these activities can generate a representative slice of the system's 'history'. Different computer runs can be used to assess the likely effects on system performance of any changes under consideration.

Another strand of OR endeavours to overcome the limitations of the classical tools to well defined problems with copious data by making use of individuals' subjective inputs. This group of methods may be described as 'intermediate'. The inputs could include expert judgements as to the likelihood and timing of uncertain future developments, or the interactions that produce system performance, or the weighting to be placed on different aspects when evaluating that performance. The model or method manipulates these quantitative inputs to produce quantitative outputs.

Thus, a system dynamics model can be used to represent complex systems which involve feedback and time-lags, and can be constructed in a participative way using the knowledge and judgement of those who have extensive experience of the system. The model can be used to predict the behaviour of the system under different conditions. The Delphi technique, by contrast, is a way of generating consensus among a group of experts in a particular field about future developments. In successive cycles, members of the

Classical	• simulation • linear programming • queuing theory • stock control • spreadsheets
Intermediate	• system dynamics • decision analysis • Delphi
New Wave	• problem structuring methods • scenario planning

Figure 10.1 Representative operational research tools and methods

group are circulated with their own most recent estimates in conjunction with the overall group response, and given the opportunity of modifying the former.

More recently there has been a development of what may be termed the 'new wave' of OR methods. These have also made use of subjective (and usually non-quantitative) inputs, and are designed for use with groups incorporating multiple perspectives. Characteristically they are deployed not for 'backroom' analysis but in facilitated workshops. The methods function by offering back to managers (perhaps with other stakeholders) a structured version of the situation in which they jointly need to make progress, with the intention of enhancing their understanding of it, it can be valuable in providing a common basis for committment.

Prominent among the new wave is the family known as problem structuring methods (PSMs). Strategic Options Development and Analysis (SODA) is one of these, and its principal technique is cognitive mapping. The approach involves eliciting from each member of a group the concepts through which they understand a problem, and the cause/effect relationships between them. This is graphically represented as a 'map' of concepts and links. These maps are merged to form a group map, to stimulate and shape workshop discussion. Cognitive mapping can also be used in conjunction with other PSMs, or even as a way of preparing for a study using classical OR tools.

Robustness analysis is also a member of the family of PSMs. It may be employed when high levels of uncertainty make the consequences of decisions hard to predict. It provides a method for evaluating alternative initial commitments in terms of the useful flexibility they leave open for future decisions. This method can be used in conjunction with projection of alternative future scenarios of the environment of the system under study; in the 'back room' mode of classical OR; or via a participative workshop in which information is elicited from group members.

Another PSM is Soft Systems Methodology. It is a generalised method of system design and re-design, which assumes that distinctive and contrasting world-views are held in relation to any significant human activity system. Participants build ideal-type conceptual models of the activities which would be necessary to operate a number of possible systems, each of which would be highly relevant from one of the world-views. They compare these models with perceptions of the existing system in order to generate debate about what changes are both culturally feasible and systemically desirable.

These approaches are commonly arrayed along a spectrum from 'hard' (classical) to 'soft' (new wave), though in reality they are distinguished from each other on more than one dimension.

It should be evident from this discussion that, in general, operational research in health services applications is close to economic evaluation (see Chapter 7). Yet, as we shall see, there is also a relevant boundary with action research (Chapter 11). This can be revealed by exploring the question, raised in the opening paragraph of this chapter, of in what sense or senses operational research can be considered to be *research*. To tackle this question we need to consider a number of very different types of OR practice.

Operational researchers may work at the improvement of tools and methods quite independently of the context of application. Or, at the other extreme, they may engage with the complex messiness of particular entangled delivery systems, with a view to illuminating key implications of possible managerial interventions – in effect a species of consultancy.

However, operational research into the substantive problems of health care delivery can be more than consultancy. This occurs, for example, when the system under study is replicated, in broad character though not in contextual detail, around a country or internationally. Under these conditions, either the particular policy adopted at the original research site, or the computer models of delivery systems on which that policy was based, can serve as a starting-point for analyses at other locations. Indeed, this use of modelling can provide a more sophisticated way of thinking about and delivering 'best practice'. It recognises that what is demonstrably 'best' in a demonstration project will not be uniformly appropriate elsewhere. Rather than 'rolling out' the policy and practice developed in a demonstration project as a standard package, modelling permits the customising of a generic framework of care for the unique local conditions existing elsewhere.

Broadly speaking, when the intention behind modelling and analysis is to produce locally useful knowledge (that is, results which the managers of the system under study find helpful), operational research is operating in consultancy mode. If, alternatively, a study is made purely with the intention of advancing knowledge about general tendencies in the management and operation of systems, then it must clearly be classified as research. However, instances of this mode specific to health care are quite rare – pure 'research' in operational research is predominantly concerned with the improvement of solutions for general types of mathematically formulated problems, which apply independently of any particular problem context. The third possibility, discussed above, is that a study is conducted with a view both to supplying decision support to the managers of a particular local system, and simultaneously generating knowledge of more general applicability. This can occur whether the method employed is classical, intermediate or new wave. OR then takes on some of the character of Action Research (see Chapter 11).

Uses

The distinctive feature of OR is modelling the relation between action and consequence. A model can be described as a simplified but consistent picture of reality, useful for thinking clearly about a problem and for trying alternative ideas.[1] Modelling can be applied in either quantitative or qualitative modes. Models in which the representations are quantitative can be used for:

- *optimisation*, in which the setting of those factors under the control of the decision-makers which can be predicted to give the most highly valued performance is identified
- *option scanning*, in which the outcomes of following a number of different decision policies of interest are predicted and compared

'Soft' models with qualitative representations may be used for:

- *problem framing*, in which the principal functions of the model are to elicit, capture and integrate separately held knowledge about the problem, in order to agree the boundaries of discussion, achieve shared understanding and facilitate mutual commitments among a heterogeneous decision-making group (in practice the 'harder' models may also be used for problem framing, but do not lend themselves so well to this interactive style of working).

Optimisation has most commonly been used in connection with routine, tactical sub-problems. When a particular practical and uncontroversial function is needed by the larger system or systems it serves, and to which it is loosely coupled, then optimisation is at its strongest. Examples might include inventory control, vehicle routing and staff rostering. The quantities of relatively good-quality data that routine, repetitive activities tend to generate (especially with the assistance of methods of automatic data capture) enable the corresponding models to be calibrated and validated with some confidence. The models can then be embedded in computer systems and used, in effect, to programme decisions (Simon 1960), so freeing up management time for other less mundane tasks.

Option scanning is generally more appropriate in situations where a change in the way in which activities are carried out is under consideration. For example, if new resources become available, it may be helpful to identify where in the current system they can most effectively be deployed. Advances in technology may present alternatives that need to be compared with current doctrine. Novel ways of delivering a service will need to be scoped in order for their viability to be assessed. The effects of actual or potential changes in organisational structure (for example, mergers or acquisitions) may need to be evaluated. For modelling work of this kind, a high degree of accuracy is neither possible (because the envisaged systems are not yet in operation) nor necessary (because broad directions of advantage rather than fine tuning are required).

The third of these modes of model-based research and practice is problem framing or structuring. This may be used in a range of different ways. Most straightforwardly, it may serve to establish the assumptions and system boundaries for quantitative modelling. However, effective problem framing can frequently produce sufficient clarification of the previously confusing tangle of complexities, uncertainties and intangibles, that no further formal analysis is sought and the way forward is clear. A more ambitious way of working is where a problem-structuring workshop is convened as a forum where representatives of different functions, departments or organisations can achieve a shared understanding of their situation. The results may range from negotiated mutual commitments through to the generation of improved alternatives for system design (Rosenhead and Mingers 2001).

With problem-structuring methods especially, the creative combination of components of different approaches is common. However, there is also scope for joint use of whole methods, or their elements, drawn more widely from the OR repertoire (Mingers and Gill 1997; Ormerod 1995; Bennett *et al.* 1997).

Given the wide variety of potential health service applications of operational research, it is hard to make general statements about their data requirements. Depending on the specifics of the situation, quantitative information may be called for on the incidence of demand and its geographical distribution, on the intensity or duration of health service activities, and on the costs associated with these activities. But there may also be a need for current or historical data on a range of social factors or behaviours which influence demand, supply, activities or costs, or for estimates of their future values.

Increasingly, data on health service activities will be drawn from routine computerised systems. Where such systems do not include key variables required by a study it may be necessary to make additional measurements. This is, however, generally a labour-intensive and lengthy procedure. Frequently the subjective estimates of expert or experienced staff are relied on to supply missing information. Thus the categories of patient incorporated in the AIDSPLAN model (see Box 10.1) were not those employed by the hospital records system. Consultants and other staff of the collaborating clinic provided experience-based estimates of health service resource inputs which distinguished between the model's categories of patients.

Box 10.1 AIDSPLAN

In the late 1980s HIV/AIDS was still a recent and poorly understood phenomenon. Particular hospitals, especially in central London, had become centres of expertise. However, elsewhere in Britain there was relatively little specialist knowledge, and considerable uncertainty about how the developing epidemic would affect other localities.

A spreadsheet model of the resources needed to treat HIV/AIDS patients was developed, based on fieldwork carried out at St Mary's Hospital, which was currently treating some 18 per cent of the national total of AIDS patients. A spreadsheet model is one of the most widely used computer applications. It enables simple bookkeeping to be carried out between the rows and columns of a two-dimensional array of data. To develop the model it was necessary to:

1   identify appropriate patient categories
2   identify resources that contributed to the treatment of people with HIV and AIDS
3   establish care options consisting of particular combinations of resources for each patient category
4   specify resource costs to turn these into costed care options

Such modelling is heavily dependent on expert medical inputs. For example, patient categories should be such that resource usage is similar within categories and different between categories. In practice this meant that these categories were defined by a rather complex combination of the following: stage of progression of the disease; adult or child status; injecting drug user or not; home circumstances.

HIV/AIDS is characterised by periods of hospitalisation alternating with care in the community. Therefore the range of resource providers was found to be wide, involving not only hospital and community health care budgets, but also the relevant local authority departments, as well as the voluntary sector. Estimates of the quantities of resources consumed were extracted from clinical records and other data bases. This enabled a set of care options to be constructed that described current practice at St Mary's Hospital.

The model had two main uses: exploring the consequences of a change of practice; and enabling 'novice' health authorities to gain some appreciation of the consequences of HIV/AIDS for their plans by inserting a range of forecasts of possible numbers in each patient category. In addition, the Department of Health incorporated a forecasting module into the software to provide estimates of suggested future patient loads.

(Rizakou et al. 1991)

Routinely collected data generally play a greater role in tactical or efficiency studies – and are highly desirable for optimisation approaches, and option scanning by computer simulation. However, the more strategic the impulse behind the study, the greater will be the reliance either on specially commissioned data collection or on expert estimates. Thus, in the Ottawa-Carleton project (see Box 10.2), a survey of service providers, users and pressure groups was conducted in order to generate a wide set of ideas about possible services which were not currently being delivered.

Box 10.2 Regional planning of health services

The Ottawa-Carleton Regional District Health Council (OCRDHC) was the largest of twenty-two district health councils established by the Ontario provincial government in the 1970s to coordinate the development of local health services. The councils' remit was solely to make recommendations to the Ministry of Health, with no independent power of implementation. OCRDHC received additional funding for a demonstration project to develop a methodology for planning for 'the availability of integrated, comprehensive health services in the region'.

Rather than attempt to draw up a ten-year or twenty-year comprehensive master plan for the region's health services, the planning team's approach was for the emerging shape of the health care system to develop through incremental changes. These changes were planned both to respond to the needs of the community, and to be shaped by a developing framework of council strategic guidelines, procedures and policies. Just three illustrations of aspects of this revised focus can be given here.

1   The methodology sought to start by 'identifying pressures for change to the health care system'. To this end, over 300 agencies which had some mandate for the delivery of health services in the region were surveyed – both to identify current provision, and to generate proposals for improvement. The approach was thus 'bottom-up' rather than 'top-down'.

2   Another key emphasis was the recognition of uncertainty as a key player. A substantial panel of experts was recruited for a Delphi exercise on the future of health care in the region. Conventional Delphis aim to generate a consensus view of the future among participants. However, in this case after giving their first round of responses, panellists were clustered into groups according to their propensity to agree on *different* futures for the health care system. In this way Delphi was adapted to generate a range of alternative perspectives on the future, rather than a single consensus view.

3   With the acceptance that certainty about the future context of the region's health systems was unattainable, the emphasis shifted away from the planning horizon towards the implementation of initial action sets. By reference to the alternative futures, it was possible to identify which of the suggested changes to the system were 'robust' – that is, kept open productive avenues of development across all the futures. This approach kept short-term gains in tension with longer-term plans.

(Best *et al.* 1986)

Those conducting an OR study should not, of course, treat data purely as necessary inputs to a model whose format is already decided upon. The data may reveal the need for a different formulation, or even the recasting of the problem to be worked on.

How to undertake operational research

The specific application of the methods of OR to questions of health service delivery now has a history of nearly fifty years. Celebrated milestones include Bailey's (1952) work on patient queues for medical care, and work by the Institute for Operational Research, part of the Tavistock Institute, on hospitals as systems (Luck *et al.* 1971). The state of OR work on health a decade later was surveyed by Boldy (1981).

A relatively recent, USA-oriented survey was reported by Pierskalla and Brailer (1994). They classified some 200 publications under the headings of system design and planning, management of operations, and medical management. The first two categories fall clearly within the scope of the delivery and organisation of health services, and include the sub-categories listed in Figure 10.2, in each case with some illustrative examples drawn from the same article.

However, by no means all of the papers covered by this survey report work carried out in conjunction with health service decision makers with the mutual intention of guiding action. The others describe analytic formulations which are *in principle* capable of representing aspects of health service organisation and delivery, but for which evidence of application is missing.

A review of practically applied modelling work in the UK (Cropper and Forte 1997) includes planning the balance of care services for elderly people, activity and capacity planning in an acute hospital, capital investment appraisal for community services, decision support for the GP consultation and the primary health care team, planning continuity of midwifery services, queue management at outpatient clinics, and preparing for a hospital's review of strategic direction.

Other recent examples of such practical work covers a wide range of health service delivery issues. These include community health needs assessment (Butler *et al.* 1995), appointments systems and functioning of outpatient clinics (Liu and Liu 1998; Taylor and Kuljis 1998), hospital capacity planning (Gove and Hewett 1995), waiting times for elective

Planning and strategy	• regional provision of specialist services
	• number and location of blood banks
	• effect on demand of opening or closing facilities
Location selection	• location of neighbourhood clinics
	• siting of emergency medical services
Capacity planning	• bed capacity and allocation between specialities
	• theatre capacity and scheduling policies
	• waiting list management
Patient scheduling	• appointments systems for outpatient clinics
	• scheduling of elective admissions, transfers, discharges
Workforce planning and scheduling	• nurse staffing – shift schedules
	• congestion and resource utilisation studies

Figure 10.2 Illustrative examples of health modelling

surgery (Martin and Smith 1995), scheduling of theatre suites (McAleer *et al.* 1995), and monitoring the performance of cardiac surgeons (Lovegrove *et al.* 1999).

The strength of OR in action can best be demonstrated by describing some practical examples. A good example would be Beech *et al.* (1997) on planning the continuity of midwifery services. Boxes 10.1–10.6 offer some further examples.

This quite diverse collection of case studies serves to demonstrate not only the breadth of possible applications, but also the range of available methods. AIDSPLAN (Box 10.1) makes use of a classical OR tool (spreadsheets); the ECMO and renal services examples (Boxes 10.3 and 10.4) demonstrate the use of simulation; the A&E model (Box 10.5) employs system dynamics, one of the 'intermediate' methods of OR; while the

---

Box 10.3 Simulation in the case of neonatal extra-corporeal membrane oxygenation (ECMO) in the Netherlands

ECMO temporarily takes over the function of the lungs and is beneficial in neonatal intensive care, but it has disadvantages as well as benefits, and it has generally been limited to those with a low predicted survival. This simulation was undertaken to investigate the consequences of the establishment of various numbers of ECMO facilities in the Netherlands.

A discrete event micro-simulation model was used. Several alternative scenarios were formulated to study the effects of plausible future events on the number of ECMO facilities required. It was estimated that between thirty-nine and fifty-six ECMO treatments would be required per year, and that the numbers of patients who might need to be treated outside the country would vary, depending on both the number of facilities and the numbers of babies born requiring treatment at any one time.

The authors state that proper planning for ECMO is particularly important because the patients cannot be put on a waiting list. The model was used to consider the problems both of over-capacity and of under-capacity, and it was concluded that an increase to fifty-six patients per year could take place without an increase in the number of ECMO facilities.

(Michel *et al.* 1996)

> **Box 10.4 Planning resources for renal services in the UK using simulation**
>
> Patients with end-stage renal failure undergo three main types of therapy: haemodialysis, continuous ambulatory peritoneal dialysis and kidney transplant. This research was undertaken to find out how many patients would require treatment in the future, of what kind, and what resources would be needed in the UK. The researchers used discrete event simulation to model patient flows through treatment.
>
> The results of the simulation showed that the number of people requiring treatment was likely to increase by 50–100 per cent over the next twenty years, and that most of these people would require dialysis. It also became clear that numbers needing treatment would vary considerably in different parts of the country, and would also vary depending on survival rates. Simulation was shown to provide a valuable way of evaluating patient numbers and flows and hence resources needs.
>
> (Davies and Roderick 1998)

Regional Planning and Paediatric Audit studies (Boxes 10.2 and 10.6) use problem-structuring methods (robustness analysis and cognitive mapping).

The studies were each designed to assist particular decision makers. However, they were also capable of generating knowledge with a wider sphere of application, and in some cases this broader focus was built into the study's remit. The motivation for the project to develop the AIDSPLAN model (Box 10.1) and to populate it with data based on practice at St Mary's Hospital in London, was to disseminate to health authorities across the UK a practical HIV/AIDS planning tool. The regional planning exercise in Ottawa-Carleton (Box 10.2) was part of a demonstration project to establish a viable planning approach for other district health councils in Ontario. And the work with the paediatric audit group (Box 10.6), apart from its potential for other audit groups, was also seen as a vehicle for the UK Department of Health's OR group to gain experience in the use of problem-structuring methods.

> **Box 10.5 Accident and emergency departments**
>
> Concern is frequently expressed about extended waits in accident and emergency (A&E) units for patients before they can be admitted as hospital inpatients. This study aimed to explore the factors underlying

and causing these unacceptable delays. The work started in conjunction with a community-based pressure group that was monitoring waiting times at all London's acute hospitals. Subsequently it developed into a collaboration with one London teaching hospital.

Many factors have been suggested as potentially responsible for these long waits, including: shortage of acute beds (both directly, and because delay caused by cancellation of scheduled operations may generate an emergency admission); behavioural responses by GPs and patients to the difficulty of gaining admission through the referrals procedure; lack of availability of acute beds because they are occupied by patients fit for discharge but without community care resources to receive them; and government waiting list initiatives which prioritise those who have waited longest, which can give precedence to less serious cases. The model was developed to contribute to this debate.

Given the prevalence of feedback loops in the situation, it was modelled using system dynamics. The flows between the community, the A&E department and the wards were each represented as rates that were subject to modification through interaction with other parts of the system. The logic of the model, as well as the quantification of its relationships, was developed through access to the hospital's data systems as well as the expertise and experience of the staff of the A&E department. The model was organised to print out the values of key performance indicators, such as the average time taken to reach different stages of the admission process, the percentage of cancellations of elective procedures, the average bed occupancy level, and the level of A&E doctor utilisation.

The effect on these indicators of running the model with different levels of demand and different bed numbers could be studied, and gave rise to some findings which appeared likely to apply not just to this one hospital. For example:

- Bed reductions result in sharp increases in elective cancellations, rather than increased waiting times in A&E.
- Increase in emergency demand by even a small percentage results in system collapse, with A&E doctors (rather than beds) the first element to be overwhelmed.
- There is insufficient slack in the system to handle random shocks.
- Hospitals are complex systems and cannot be managed effectively by using any single measure as the touchstone for performance.

(Lane et al. 2000)

In the other projects, some significant outputs emerged which were not part of the original research design. Thus the A&E study (Box 10.5) was designed to develop a tool for exploring the interconnections that drive waiting times. However, it generated insights in a number of other areas, including the role of performance indicators in policy steering.

Box 10.6 Paediatric audit

In the early 1990s the British government made medical audit mandatory for doctors. A number of bodies sponsored a study of whether and how problem structuring methods (PSMs) could assist audit. Medical audit is the systematic critical analysis by health service staff of the quality of medical care that they deliver. This is a group activity, involving members of the speciality group with very different roles. Furthermore, audit was a sensitive topic, with some doctors resentful of this 'distraction' from direct patient care. So an approach which sought to elicit individual perspectives as a means of developing shared commitments at a group meeting seemed potentially appropriate. PSMs in general are designed for work with groups, and Strategic Operations Development and Analysis (SODA) (Eden and Ackermann 2001) in particular is a member of the PSM family with the desired characteristics. There was also an abbreviated deployment of Soft Systems Methodology.

The work was carried out with the paediatric specialty group at a district hospital which was about to embark on audit for the first time. Ten members were involved, in the categories of consultant, registrar, junior doctor, nurse, manager and audit clerk. Each member of the group was interviewed separately, and a cognitive map of his or her thinking about audit (the concepts in use and the cause/effect relations between them) was elicited. These maps were then combined into a merged map, with links provided by the concepts repeated in more than one map.

The merged map provided the structure for a discussion at a meeting of the whole group. Various aspects were singled out for attention (including some which had been generated by junior members who might have been unwilling to vocalise those same remarks in front of their seniors). Some commitments were made about both the process and the topics for the future practice of audit by the group. According to the Audit Officer for the hospital, this group achieved the fastest 'take-off' into audit of all the groups for which she was responsible.

(Gains and Rosenhead 1993)

Limitations

Given the diverse problems that OR can address, the identification of the limits of its sphere of activity is not straightforward. Evidently excluded are those managerial issues which are the exclusive domains of well defined technical specialisms (though there are some contestable boundaries, notably with economics). Broadly, issues in which either complexity or uncertainty or both are central are likely to be well served by OR approaches. The addition to this brew of multiple agencies with potential conflicts between them indicates the potential applicability of problem structuring methods.

Some apparent limitations of operational research arise from the selection and use of inappropriate methods from the OR repertoire. The most high-profile example of this is the Balance of Care Model, perhaps the most expensive OR project in UK civilian government history. It was conceived as an aid to strategic decision making on the level of provision (either nationally or locally) of resources for institutional and community care, and for the allocation of care groups between these modes. However, it was cast as an optimisation problem, and three successive versions were developed in an attempt to persuade decision makers to use it. It started as a complex model; the second version was more complex still; and the third version tried to separate out the optimisation and option scanning functions – all virtually to no avail (Boldy *et al.* 1981; Rosenhead 1984; Smith 1995). Finally all vestiges of optimisation were removed and it became a pure option scanning tool (in fact, a spreadsheet model), and became modestly useful (Forte and Bowen 1997). This final version was the direct ancestor of the AIDSPLAN model described in Box 10.1. Provided tools and methods are matched to problem situations, the diversity of operational research now makes it potentially valuable across a broad range.

Other limitations on the use of OR for health service delivery and organisation may arise from the organisational arrangements for its provision – and these inevitably differ from country to country. However, in the UK at this time, perhaps the major current limitation on the use of OR is its relatively weak institutionalisation as a discipline within the operational levels of the health services.

Acknowledgements

I am extremely grateful for advice and information received in the preparation of this chapter from Gwyn Bevan, Paul Forte, Penny Mullen, Diane Plamping, Geoff Royston and Peter Smith.

Note

1   I am grateful to my colleague John Howard for this formulation.

Further reading

Operational research

Pidd, M. (1996) *Tools for Thinking*, Chichester: Wiley.

Problem structuring methods

Rosenhead, J. (ed.) (1989) *Rational Analysis for a Problematic World: Problem Structuring Methods for Complexity, Uncertainty and Conflict*, Chichester: Wiley (revised edn edited by J. Rosenhead and J. Mingers to be published in 2001).

Applications of OR to health service problems and issues

Cropper, S. and Forte, P. (eds) (1997) *Enhancing Health Services Management: the Role of Decision Support Systems*, Buckingham: Open University Press.
Matson, E. (ed.) (1997) *Operational Research Applied to Health Services*, Trondheim: Norwegian Institute of Science and Technology.

Applications of OR to one complex problem area

Kaplan, E. H. and Brandeau, M. L. (eds) (1994) *Modelling the AIDS Epidemic: Planning, Policy and Prediction*, New York: Raven Press.

Contextualisation of the contribution of OR within tendencies in health care

Royston, G. (1998) 'Shifting the balance of care into the 21st century', *European Journal of Operational Research*, 105: 267–76.

For ongoing material, see the journal *Health Care Management Science*.

References

Bailey, N. T. J. (1952) 'A study of queues and appointment systems in hospital outpatient departments', *Journal of the Royal Statistical Society*, 14: 185–99.
Beech, R., Mejia, A. and Shirazi, R. (1997) 'A decision support system for planning continuity of midwifery services', in S. Cropper and P. Forte (eds) *Enhancing Health Services Management: The Role of Decision Support Systems*, 165–76, Buckingham: Open University Press.
Bennett, P., Ackermann, F., Eden, C. and Williams, T. (1997) 'Analysing litigation and negotiation: using a combined methodology', in J. Mingers and A. Gill (eds) *Multimethodology: The Theory and Practice of Combining Methodologies*, 59–88, Chichester: Wiley.
Best, G., Parston, G. and Rosenhead, J. (1986) 'Robustness in practice: the regional planning of health services', *Journal of the Operational Research Society*, 37: 463–78.
Boldy, D. (ed.) (1981) *Operational Research Applied to Health Services*, London: Croom Helm.

Boldy, D., Canvin, R., Russell, J. and Royston, G. (1981) 'Planning the balance of care', in D. Boldy (ed.) *Operational Research Applied to Health Services*, 84–108, London: Croom Helm.

Butler, T., Sparks, C. and Oxley, D. (1995) 'Community health needs assessment', *OR Insight*, 8, 3: 2–8.

Cropper, S. and Forte, P. (1997) *Enhancing Health Services Management: The Role of Decision Support Systems*, Buckingham: Open University Press.

Davies, R. and Roderick, P. (1998) 'Planning resources for renal services throughout UK using simulation', *European Journal of Operational Research*, 105: 285–95.

Eden, C. and Ackermann, F. (2001) 'SODA – the principles', in J. Rosenhead and J. Mingers (eds) *Rational Analysis for a Problematic World Revisited: Problem Structuring Methods for Complexity, Uncertainty and Conflict*, 21–42, Chichester: Wiley.

Forte, P. and Bowen, T. (1997) 'Improving the balance of elderly care services', in S. Cropper and P. Forte (eds) *Enhancing Health Services Management: The Role of Decision Support Systems*, 71–85, Buckingham: Open University Press.

Gains, A. and Rosenhead, J. (1993) 'Problem structuring for medical quality assurance', Working Paper 93.8, Operational Research, London School of Economics.

Gove, D. and Hewett, D. (1995) 'A hospital capacity planning model', *OR Insight*, 8, 2: 12–15.

Lane, D. C., Mondefeldt, C. and Rosenhead, J. (2000) 'Looking in the wrong place for healthcare improvements: a system dynamics study of an accident and emergency department', *Journal of the Operational Research Society*, 51: 518–31.

Liu, L. and Liu, X. (1998) 'Block appointment systems for outpatient clinics with multiple doctors', *Journal of the Operational Research Society*, 49: 1254–9.

Lovegrove, J., Sherlaw-Johnson, C., Valencia, O., Treasure T. and Gallivan, S. (1999) 'Monitoring the performance of cardiac surgeons', *Journal of the Operational Research Society*, 50: 684–9.

Luck, G. M., Luckman, J., Smith, B. W. and Stringer, J. (1971) *Patients, Hospitals and Operational Research*, London: Tavistock.

McAleer, W. E., Turner, J. A., Lismore, D. and Nagui, I. A. (1995) 'Simulation of a hospital's theatre suite', *Journal of Management in Medicine*, 9, 5: 14–26.

Martin, S. and Smith, P. (1995) *Modelling Waiting Times for Elective Surgery*, York: Centre for Health Economics, University of York.

Michel, B. C., van Staveren, R. J. E., Geven, W. B. and van Hout, B. A. (1996) 'Simulation models in the planning of health care facilities: an application in the case of neonatal extracorporeal membrane oxygenation', *Journal of Health Services Research and Policy*, 1: 198–204.

Mingers, J. and Gill, A. (eds) (1997) *Multimethodology: The Theory and Practice of Combining Methodologies*, Chichester: Wiley.

Ormerod, R. (1995) 'Putting soft OR methods to work: information systems development at Sainsbury's supermarkets', *Journal of the Operational Research Society*, 46: 277–93.

Pierskalla, W. P. and Brailer, D. J. (1994) 'Applications of operations research in health care delivery', in S. M. Pollock, M. H. Rothkopf and A. Barnett (eds) *Operations Research in the Public Sector*, 469–505, Amsterdam: Elsevier.

Rizakou, E., Rosenhead, J. and Reddington, K. (1991) 'AIDSPLAN: a decision support model for planning the provision of HIV/AIDS-related services', *Interfaces*, 21: 117–29.

Rosenhead, J. (1984) 'Operational research in social planning', in J. Midgley and D. Piachaud (eds) *The Fields and Methods of Social Planning*, 147–76, London: Heinemann.

Rosenhead, J. and Mingers, J. (eds) (2001) *Rational Analysis for a Problematic World Revisited: Problem Structuring Methods for Complexity, Uncertainty and Conflict*, Chichester: Wiley.

Simon, H. A. (1960) *The New Science of Management Decision*, New York: Harper and Row.

Smith, P. (1995) 'Large scale models and large scale thinking: the case of health services', *Omega*, 8: 145–57.

Taylor, S. and Kuljis, J. (1998) 'Simulation in health care management: modelling an outpatient clinic', *OR Insight*, 11, 3: 7–11.

Chapter 11

Action research

Julienne Meyer

Introduction

This chapter begins by defining action research in terms of its theoretical basis and describing its three key elements: participatory character, democratic impulse, and simultaneous contribution to social science and social change. Next it outlines how action research can be used and describes its different forms in practice. It considers its overlap with other methods and highlights its use in studying the delivery and organisation of health services. Given that action research is an approach and not a unique discipline or method, only brief mention is made of the methods used. Finally, the limitations of action research are addressed by considering its validity, the danger of exploiting participants, the difficulties of generalising from the results, and the challenge of developing theory.

Definition and theoretical basis

Action research is an approach to research rather than a unique discipline or a particular method. It has been in existence for over fifty years (Lewin 1946) and has become associated with a variety of definitions and uses in a wide range of areas (e.g. group dynamics, organisational change, community development, education and nursing). Action research has changed over time in response to emergent methodological debates, which have seen a movement from positivist and interpretivist approaches (see Chapter 1) to more collaborative ways of generating knowledge (Meyer 1993). As such, action research has come to be seen as part of a new paradigm of research (Reason and Rowan 1981), which emphasises the need to do research *with* and *for* people rather than *on* them. Throughout the literature the term is used loosely, and no one definition captures the range of meanings. However, Eden and Huxham (1996) assert that, in relation to the study of organisations, 'Action research involves the researcher in working with members of an organisation over a matter which is of genuine concern to them and in which there is an intent by the organisation members to take action based on the intervention'.

Essentially, action research is concerned with generating knowledge about a social system while, at the same time, attempting to change it. Unlike the other forms of research discussed in this book, which focus on generating findings that later may, or may not, be implemented in practice, action research focuses on changing practice as part of the research process itself. Its strength lies in its focus on generating solutions to practical problems and its ability to empower practitioners, managers and users to engage with research and development activities. Participants can choose to research their own practice, or an outside researcher can be engaged to help them identify problems, seek and implement practical solutions, and systematically monitor and reflect on the process and outcome of change. Throughout the study, findings are fed back to participants to inform decisions about the next stage of the study. This formative style of research is thus responsive to events as they naturally occur in the field, and frequently entails collaborative spirals of planning, acting, observing, reflecting, and replanning.

Reports of action research need to take account of the social, historical and political dimensions of the practice that is being changed. This is particularly useful in the study of organisations, which need to take account of whole systems in their broad context. The action researcher writes their own interpretation of events, and those being studied (users, carers, professionals) have access to these accounts. They are able to comment critically on them and ensure that their own accounts are also represented. In this way action research values multiple accounts. It tries to capture the realities of everyday practice and report findings in context, so that the reader might judge the relevance of the findings to their own particular situation. Action research accepts that reality exists independently of the researcher's claims about it, and that those claims may be more or less accurate, depending on their context. It represents the middle way, described by Hammersley (1992) as 'subtle realism' (see Chapter 1 in this volume), which seeks to represent reality while recognising that phenomena can be represented from different perspectives.

There are various different forms of action research, which have emerged in response to methodological debates in different disciplines. Hart and Bond (1995) have devised a typology (Table 11.1) which distinguishes four types: experimental, organisational, professionalising and empowering, in relation to seven distinguishing criteria. The 'experimental' type is best characterised by Lewin's change experiments and his concern to discover general laws of social life to inform policy-making (Lewin 1946). The 'organisational' type represents the application of action research to organisational problem solving, and has its core in overcoming resistance to change and creating more productive relationships. The 'professionalising' type is informed by an agenda grounded in practice, characterised by the new professions keen to develop research-based practice, e.g. nursing, teaching, social work. Finally, the 'empowering' type is most commonly associated

Table 11.1 Action research typology

Action Research type: distinguishing criteria	Consensus model of society / Rational social management		Conflict model of society / Structural change	
	Experimental	Organisational	Professionalising	Empowering
1 Educative Base	Re-education — Enhancing social science administrative control and social change towards consensus	Re-education training — Enhancing managerial control and organisational change towards consensus	Reflective practice — Enhancing professional control and individual's ability to control work situation	Consciousness-raising — Enhancing user-control and shifting balance of power; structural change towards pluralism
	Inferring relationship between behaviour and output; identifying causal factors in group dynamics	Overcoming resistance to change restructuring balance of power between managers and workers	Empowering professional groups; advocacy on behalf of patients clients	Empowering oppressed groups
	Social scientific bias researcher focused	Managerial bias client-focused	Practitioner focused	User practitioner-focused
2 Individuals in groups	Closed group, controlled, selection made by researcher for purposes of measurement inferring relationship between cause and effect	Work groups and/or mixed groups of managers and workers	Professional(s) and/or (interdisciplinary) professional group negotiated team boundaries	Fluid groupings, self selecting or natural boundary or open/closed by negotiation
	Fixed membership	Selected membership	Shifting membership	Fluid membership
3 Problem focus	Problem emerges from the interaction of social science theory and social problems	Problem defined by most powerful group; some negotiation with workers	Problem defined by professional group; some negotiation with users	Emerging and negotiated definition of problem by less powerful group(s)
	Problem relevant for social science management interests	Problem relevant for management/social science interests	Problem emerges from professional practice experience	Problem emerges from members' practice experience
	Success defined in terms of social science	Success defined by sponsors	Contested, professionally determined definitions of success	Competing definitions of success accepted and expected

4 Change intervention	Social science experimental intervention to test theory or generate theory	Top-down, directed change towards predetermined aims	Professionally led, predefined, process-led	Bottom-up, undetermined, process-led
	Problem to be solved in terms of research aims	Problem to be solved in terms of management aims	Problem to be resolved in the interests of research-based practice and professionalisation	Problem to be explored as part of the process of change, developing an understanding of meanings of issues in terms of problem and solution
5 Improvement and involvement	Towards controlled outcome and consensual definition of improvement	Towards tangible outcome and consensual definition of improvement	Towards improvement in practice defined by professionals and on behalf of others	Towards negotiated outcomes and pluralist definitions of improvement: account taken of vested interest
6 Cyclic processes	Research components dominant	Action and research components in tension; action dominated	Research and action components in tension; research-dominated	Action components dominant
	Identifies causal processes that can be generalised	Identifies causal processes that are specific to problem context and/or can be generalised	Identifies causal processes that are specific to problem and/or can be generalised	Change course of events; recognition of multiple influences upon change
	Time limited, task focused	Discrete cycles, rationalist, sequential	Spiral of cycle, opportunistic, dynamic	Open-ended, process-driven
7 Research relationship, degree of collaboration	Experimenter respondents	Consultant researcher, respondent participants	Practitioner or researcher collaborators	Practitioner researcher co-researchers co-change agents
	Outside researcher as expert research funding	Client pays an outside consultant – 'they who pay the piper, call the tune'	Outside resources and/or internally generated	Outside resources and/or internally generated
	Differentiated roles	Differential roles	Merged roles	Shared roles

Source: Hart and Bond 1995: 40–3

with community development approaches, and is characterised by an explicit anti-oppressive stance to working with vulnerable groups in society.

While this typology is useful to understand the complexities of action research, its multidimensional nature means that it is not easy to classify individual studies (Meyer 2000). This makes choosing the right approach to action research problematic. While particular individuals may have ideological leanings towards one type or other, it is important to choose an approach that best suits the context of the study. Somekh (1994) notes the effect of occupational cultures upon action research methodology, and supports the notion that its definition should be grounded in the values and discourse of the individual or group being studied, rather than in any particular methodological school of thought. Whichever approach is taken, the action researcher needs to be explicit about their intended approach, and to have negotiated this with participants in advance of the study. Funders need to be persuaded that the proposed approach will gather appropriate data to give insights into the subject of the study.

According to Carr and Kemmis (1986), most definitions of action research incorporate three important elements: its participatory character, its democratic impulse, and its simultaneous contribution to social science and social change.

Participatory character

Participation is fundamental to action research. Action research is carried out by people directly concerned with the social situation that is being researched, and is concerned with the practical questions arising in their everyday work (Elliott 1991). A precondition of action research is that participants perceive a need to initiate change and are willing to engage with research to scrutinise their work. Action researchers recognise that change is more effective when brought about by the voluntary participation of those involved, rather than when it is imposed autocratically from above. Furthermore, they believe that research studies are best designed in the context of their application, in collaboration with those who will ultimately be responsible for implementing interventions to be evaluated. Thus action research requires a different level of commitment from participants than more traditional studies, and the clear-cut demarcation between the 'researcher' and 'researched' is blurred.

It is important to note that action research is responsive to participants' needs and it is therefore not possible, at the outset, to determine the details of the study. Thus informed consent cannot be gained in the traditional way, but must be continually negotiated throughout. Instead, consideration must be given to establishing an ethical framework within which to conduct the research. For instance, participants need to feel that they can withdraw from the study at any time, and that they have some control and ownership of the data and how these are shared with a wider audience. Change can be threatening and, in advance of the study, participants should have some say in how the situation should be managed if tensions arise.

Democratic impulse

Action research is concerned with an intervention to bring about change and improvement (Elliott 1991). The democratic impulse in an action research study, within health care settings, is not only concerned with empowering professionals to systematically examine and change their practice, but also with empowering lay people to be more in control of their health care. As Blaxter (1995) notes, it is an approach ideally suited to the involvement of users and carers in research and development. The empowerment which action research produces is significant, as it is concerned with bringing about change. By working collaboratively with participants, it is possible to uncover contradictions and conflicts that stand in the way of change. Participants in action research are empowered to address issues that have previously been hidden and, through this process of enlightenment, are given the opportunity to influence change. Furthermore, through working closely with participants, it is possible to gain insight into the constraints of the everyday practices that impose limits on what can be achieved in terms of change. It is thus a very useful approach to understand better some of the contradictions between health care policy and practice. 'Democracy' in action research usually requires participants to be seen as equals. The researcher works as a facilitator of change, consulting with participants not only on the action process but also on how it will be evaluated. Throughout the study, findings are fed back to participants for validation and to inform decisions about the next stage of the study. This requires excellent interpersonal skills as well as research skills. Frequently, action researchers are working across traditional boundaries (for example, health and social care, hospital and community settings, management and practice) and need to be able to juggle different and competing agendas.

Simultaneous contribution to social science and social change

A strength of action research is its ability to influence practice positively while simultaneously gathering data to share with a wider audience. Its eclectic use of methods for data collection requires researchers to have a broad understanding of social sciences. Action research is often written up as a case study (Yin 1994). As with all case study research, a multi-method approach to data collection (for instance, field notes, interviews, structured instruments, documentary evidence) is frequently taken, which allows for the triangulation of data (Jick 1979). Triangulation involves looking at the same phenomenon from a variety of approaches, with a view to verifying findings (see Chapter 1). This can often lead to some interesting insights, especially when the findings do not support each other (Meyer 1995).

Action researchers also need to have good facilitation skills for bringing about change. However, it should be noted that change is often problematic, and although action research lends itself well to the discovery of solutions, its success should not be judged solely in terms of the size of change achieved or the immediate implementation of solutions. Success should also be viewed in relation to what has been learnt from the experience of undertaking the work. For instance, a study (Meyer and Bridges 1998; Bridges *et al.* 2000) that set out to explore the care of older people in an A&E department did not result in much change in the course of the study. However, the lessons learnt from the research were reviewed in the context of national policy and other research findings, and carefully fed back to those working in the hospital. As a result, changes were made within the organisation based on the study's recommendations. This study was able to identify some of the special needs of older people in A&E and to identify a number of 'gaps' in care. It also achieved some positive changes (for example, specialist discharge posts were established in the A&E department) and highlighted a number of practical issues to enable debate and priority setting to take place (for project summary, see Box 11.1).

Box 11.1 An action research study into the organisation of care for older people in the Accident and Emergency department

Questions
- What is the nature of the current organisation of care for older patients in A&E?
- How do older users and carers perceive the care in A&E?
- How can improvements in received care be achieved?

Local background
- One of the busiest A&E departments in the country
- 3,592 attendances aged seventy-five and over (November 1996–February 1997)
- Mean attendance thirty older people per day
- 12.6 per cent of these patients had already been referred to hospital by a general practitioner.

Pressures for change
- Audit Commission report on A&E services, 1996

- District Audit report on services for older people with fractured neck of femur, 1995/96
- Review of the quality of training for specialist registrars, 1996
- Winter pressures on available beds, 1996/97

Methods

- Action researcher: trained as clinical nurse specialist in acute elderly care
- Multi-method – process and outcomes of change
- 'Bottom-up' approach to change
- Regular feedback of findings to plan next stage of action and/or enquiry
- Multiple perspectives (users and carers, professionals, managers)

Main action-reflection spirals

- Care while in A&E
- Discharge from A&E
- Admission to inpatient bed while in A&E

Findings

- Changes in care delivery by A&E staff, e.g. standard social history checklist for A&E nurses
- Changes in supporting structures to A&E practice, e.g. successful pilot of specialists' posts in A&E
- Other changes, e.g. reduction in strain on the capacity of A&E and inpatient wards
- Remaining gaps, e.g. assessments of pressure sore risk not routinely carried out on older patients
- Researcher's interpretations:
    organisation: 'A battleground'
    patients: 'Little things that count'
    staff: 'Disempowered to care'

Uses

It is increasingly being recognised that research evidence is not sufficiently influencing practice (Walshe *et al.* 1995) and that there is a need to focus more on the development end of the R&D spectrum. Barriers to implementing research-based practice are likely to be both organisational and individual and, in planning services, there is a need to take both perspectives into account. Action research lends itself to studying both perspectives simultaneously.

For instance, there is no point in designing services without taking account of the behaviour of individuals within the system. While it is generally accepted by proponents of the evidence-based health care movement that randomised trials are the best designs for evaluating interventions (see Chapter 4) and qualitative studies (see Chapter 3) are best for understanding patients' experiences, attitudes, and beliefs (DiCenso and Cullum 1998), it is also recognised that the findings of traditional research are not always appropriate to the needs of individual patients, and that clinical expertise and professional judgement are needed to implement findings wisely at this level (Sackett *et al.* 1997). Thus new approaches are needed, not only to explore the factors that influence the implementation of scientific evidence in practice, but also to explore the nature of professional decision making in relation to individual cases. Action research can facilitate this process and produce a new type of knowledge, namely 'craft knowledge' (Titchen 2000). In research on health service delivery and organisation, it is important to feed this knowledge into systems that are evaluating how services can be improved.

By exploring the epistemology of practice implicit in the intuitive processes that practitioners have to bring to situations of uncertainty, instability, uniqueness and value conflict (Schon 1987), a better understanding is gained of how services are delivered and how organisations need to be altered to take greater account of these behaviours. Schon (1987) maintains that in practice, through a process of reflection-in-action, practitioners cope with uncertainty by reflecting on what they are doing in a unique situation and restructuring their understanding as a result. Thus the practitioner is not dependent on the categories of established theory and technique, but constructs a new theory of the unique case. In this way, practitioners build their own personal theories, which over time cluster into experiential knowledge. Professional judgement is thought to be based on an interplay of scientific, personal and experiential knowledge. 'Practitioner-centred' approaches are considered the most appropriate means of unpacking this craft knowledge.

Rolfe (1998) identifies three methods that are practitioner-led: single case experimental designs, reflective case studies and reflexive action research. He argues that practitioners should develop research roles in their everyday practice in order to develop this practical knowledge, and suggests they have three research needs. First, he argues that practitioners should find a way to verify the findings and recommendations of scientific research in their own practice and for their own patients; second, he suggests that they need to test out personal theories in practice; third, they need to integrate practice and research in their everyday work, wherever possible.

One key issue is whether research should be undertaken by a neutral disinterested outsider, or by an insider who has a closer relationship with those being researched. The debates are inconclusive, but it is interesting to note that process evaluations in schools, where practitioners inform outside researchers about the nature of their work, have led to institutional self-evaluation with teachers being seen to be the best judges of their own practices (Simons 1981).

Action research can be used in three ways to generate different types of knowledge. It is useful:

- when no evidence exists to support or refute current practice or when poor knowledge, skills and attitudes exist to carry out evidence-based practice;
- when gaps have been identified in service provision, or services are underused or deemed inappropriate; and
- when new roles are being developed and evaluated and there is a need to work across traditional conflicting boundaries.

Box 11.2 and Box 11.3 illustrate examples of action research applied to a health service organisation and delivery question about which there is little evidence.

Box 11.2 Continuous quality improvement in an acute hospital

This action research study aimed to improve the quality of three departments within a hospital (medical records, X-ray and operating theatres) in terms of the services they provided to other departments.

The change innovation was the use of 'quality circles' whereby staff work in multidisciplinary intensive group sessions to generate ideas to improve quality.

The study collected data at the different stages of the action research cycle. For example, at the planning stage, the study describes the ideas generated by the quality circles, including developing a patient questionnaire, consultations on standard testing and an exchange visit to another hospital. The processes following these were documented by the study for each department, e.g. in the X-ray department, although staff were keen to improve quality and had many ideas, they were disorganised and no implementation of ideas was recorded. In the medical records department, the manager reported significant improvements, but no independent validation of these improvements was reported.

The authors conclude that bottom-up change strategies such as quality circles and action research strategies have more effect on staff attitudes and behaviour than a top-down approach.

(Potter et al. 1994)

Box 11.3 Evaluation of a reorganisation of acute medical care in a district general hospital.

This study concerned the conversion of six general medical wards into a thirty-eight-bed medical admission unit. The aim of the study was to describe these changes to acute medical care and assess their impact on staff and patients.

The change innovation involved the action research cycle of information gathering, planning and implementation. At each phase, health care professionals and managers were involved in the process.

The evaluation collected data on process outcomes (e.g. creation of a new medical admissions unit) and outputs such as activity data before and after interventions (e.g. number of admissions, length of stay and time from first diagnosis to consultant match). Surveys were conducted of staff and patients.

The study reported that the new unit had been established but pre- and post-intervention data reveal a mixed picture. On the positive side, the study cited evidence for improved collaboration and team approach to the care of patients, improved first diagnosis, better consultant match, and a more appropriate staff skill mix for patients' needs. Patients reported feeling more ready for discharge. However, admissions continued to rise following the intervention, medical staff reported more concern over blocked beds, and nursing staff, while reporting increased time for health promotion, also reported increased stress.

(Hanlon *et al.* 1997)

How to undertake action research

Given that action research is an approach and not a method, there is no set way to do it. It usually involves multiple research methods, most of which are qualitative, although some quantitative surveys may form part of the process (Bowling 1997). Stringer (1996) proposes that action research broadly follows the following stages: 'setting the stage', 'looking', 'thinking', and 'acting'.

During 'setting the stage', the investigator acts as a facilitator and needs to identify and involve all relevant stakeholders. The facilitators need to negotiate their role carefully with each of the stakeholder groups. In the 'looking' phase the investigator needs to describe the problem and its context. Eden and Huxham (1996) emphasise the importance of developing an explicit research process in action research, which includes aiming to draw out theory. During the 'thinking' stage, Stringer (1996) says the investigator should analyse the situation in order to develop their understanding of the problem. Finally, in the 'acting' phase, the solutions to the problem need to be planned by all the stakeholders facilitated by the investigator. The processes involved and the role of facilitator are described in detail by Stringer (1996).

Hart and Bond (1995) have compiled a 'toolkit' which they recommend for use in action research. It includes a self-assessment questionnaire designed to help with thinking about the research problem and the proposed research; groupwork guidelines such as factors the facilitator should consider, advice on starting programmes, and ethical guidelines; advice on diary-keeping for facilitators as a form of field-notes; methods for self-reflection and evaluating performance and progress; advice on evaluation (e.g. using basic records or surveys, etc.); and the use of structured attitude scales.

Given that both qualitative and quantitative methods can be used within any study, and the open-ended and responsive nature of action research, this makes it extremely difficult to identify specific criteria by which to judge the quality of action research. Instead, one needs to be guided by some underlying principles and be reassured that those engaged in action research are aware of the complexities, and have both the research and interpersonal skills with which to carry it out. Eden and Huxham (1996) specify fifteen characteristics of action research, as a checklist to guide thinking about the design and validity of studies.

Limitations

Four potential limitations of action research have been identified: difficulties in establishing the validity and reliability of the findings; the danger of exploiting participants; the challenge of generalising a single study; and the relative lack of theoretical development.

Assessing validity and reliability

In critiquing action research, care needs to be taken not to apply inappropriate arguments from a different paradigm of research. Traditional notions of validity and reliability need to be viewed from a different perspective in action research. Guba and Lincoln (1989) suggest that the techniques required are triangulation, reflexivity and member checks. First, triangulation is critical in establishing the validity of results, requiring multiple data sources, methods and theoretical schemes (see Chapter 1). By triangulating the data using multiple methods, the undue influence of a single data set and possible researcher bias are thought to be minimised. Action research also acknowledges the role of context in influencing findings, and seeks to describe the setting in its historical and socio-political context. Second, Guba and Lincoln argue the need for reflexive subjectivity in substantiating the trustworthiness of data. Self-reflective inquiry attempts to guard against the damages of being a long-term observer, such as contrivance, 'going native', research exhaustion, ethnocentrism and perceptual bias. Reflexivity also allows action researchers to justify the selection of informants when theoretical sampling (Glaser and Strauss 1967) is used, and to explain biases in the data and conclusions created by the selection of participants. Third, member checks are important in proving the trustworthiness of data. These involve recycling the categories, emerging findings, and conclusions back to at least a sample of respondents. In action research, assessing participant confirmation and reaction to findings by use of feedback and close monitoring in the field setting is thought to be instrumental in revealing researcher-induced bias.

Exploitation of participants

Action research can be seen as too idealistic. Collaborative research implies equality of relationship between researcher and participant, but it is questionable to what extent this is really possible. Stacey (1988) questions whether the greater respect for, and equality with, research subjects masks a deeper, more dangerous form of exploitation. Power relations cannot be ignored, particularly in hierarchical contexts such as health care settings. It is naive to think that gaining different stakeholder perspectives will lead to consensus and negotiated change. Action research can bring to the surface the underlying value system, including norms and conflicts, which may be at the core of problems identified. The psycho-social costs of this should not be ignored (Meyer 1993). While the researcher can withdraw at any time, participants are likely to want to remain in their chosen area of practice. Clearly, careful consideration needs to be given to the form of action research adopted. Conflict cannot be ignored, and an ethical code of practice needs to be agreed with participants before starting the study.

Generalisability of findings

Generalisations made from action research studies are different from those made from traditional research studies. Action research offers a surrogate experience and invites the reader to underwrite the account, by appealing to their tacit knowledge of human situations. The truths contained in a successful study are assumed by the shock of recognition (Carr and Kemmis 1986). Reports need to be authentic, detailed, rigorously accurate and impartial (Simons 1981). It is important to make the report accessible to both public and professional judgement. Through systematically feeding back findings throughout an action research study, it is possible to check the account with participants. However, the relevance of the findings to any other situation rests with the reader.

The generalisability of action research is often underestimated because of a fundamental confusion about two distinct logical bases upon which generalisations can be made: the empirical and the theoretical (Sharp 1998). Empirical generalisation is concerned with showing that some relevant characteristics of a sample are typical of the population. By contrast, theoretical generalisation is based on identifying some general principle concerning the phenomenon in question and seeking to explain the association. The adequacy of the theoretical explanation can be tested in relation to the extent to which it is not contradicted by other empirical observations. However, it should be noted that more than one theoretical explanation can be used to explain an association, so this in itself does not tell us whether the theory is adequate or not. Case studies, particularly when used in an action research project, are a useful means by which theoretical explanations of phenomena can be generated. In addition, findings may be applicable to other settings by the transparency of the action research process. Whatever the method of generalisation, the findings of action research should not be dismissed as mere anecdote.

Lack of theory development

Action research is sometimes criticised for its lack of theory development. The focus on action can sometimes reduce the time available to theorise more widely. However, as an approach to research, it is concerned with the learning not only of participants, but also of a wider audience. Often action research accounts are written up in the format of a case study, from which theoretical explanations can be generated without the need for empirical typicality (Hammersley *et al.* 2000). Thus case studies of action research can be used to uncover causal *processes* linking inputs and outputs within a system. However, there is also the scope for the use of comparative method in cross-case analysis of action research. Either way, the onus lies with the action researcher to develop theoretically rigorous conclusions from their studies.

Further reading

Argyris, C., Putnam, R. and McLain Smith, D. (1996) *Action Science: Concepts, Methods and Skills for Research and Intervention*, San Francisco: Jossey-Bass.

Carr, W. and Kemmis, S. (1986) *Becoming Critical: Education, Knowledge and Action Research*, London: The Falmer Press.

Eden, C. and Huxham, C. (1996) 'Action research for the study of organisations', in S. Clegg, C. Hardy and W. Nord (eds) *Handbook of Organisational Studies*, 526–42, London: Sage.

Elliot, J. (1991) *Action Research for Educational Change*, Milton Keynes: Open University Press.

Greenwood, D. and Levin, M. (1998) *Introduction to Action Research: Social Research for Social Change*, London: Sage.

Hart, E. and Bond, M. (1995) *Action Research for Health and Social Care: A Guide to Practice*, Milton Keynes: Open University Press.

McNiff, J. (2000) *Action Research and Organisations*, London: Routledge.

Reason, P. (2000) *Handbook of Action Research: Participative Inquiry and Practice*, London: Sage.

Stringer, E. T. (1996) *Action Research: A Handbook for Practitioners*, London: Sage.

Susman, G. I. and Evered, R. D. (1978) 'An assessment of the scientific merits of action research', *Administrative Science Quarterly*, 23: 582–603.

Waterman, H., Tillen, D., Dickson, R. and de Koning, K. (in preparation) *Action Research: A Systematic Review and Guidance for Assessment*, Health Technology Assessment (HTA) R&D Programme, London: Department of Health.

Winter, R. and Munn-Giddings, C. (2001) *A Handbook for Action Research in Health and Social Care*, London: Routledge.

Zuber-Skerritt, O. (ed.) (1996) *New Directions in Action Research*, London: Taylor and Francis.

References

Blaxter, M. (1995) *Consumers and Research in the NHS*, Leeds: Department of Health NHS Executive.

Bowling, A. (1997) *Research Methods in Health: Investigating Health and Health Services*, Buckingham: Open University Press.

Bridges, J., Meyer, J. and Spilsbury, K. (2000) 'Organisation of care for older people in A&E', *Emergency Nurse*, 8, 3: 22–6.

Carr, W. and Kemmis, S. (1986) *Becoming Critical: Education, Knowledge and Action Research*, London: The Falmer Press.

DiCenso, A. and Cullum, N. (1998) 'Implementing evidence-based nursing: some misconceptions', *Evidence-Based Nursing*, 1, 2: 38–40.

Eden, C. and Huxham, C. (1996) 'Action research for the study of organisations', in S. Clegg, C. Hardy and W. Nord (eds) *Handbook of Organisation Studies*, 526–42, London: Sage.

Elliott, J. (1991) *Action Research for Educational Change: Developing Teachers and Teaching*, Milton Keynes: Open University Press.

Glaser, B. G. and Strauss, A. L. (1967) *The Discovery of Grounded Theory: Strategies for Qualitative Research*, Chicago: Aldine.

Guba, Y. and Lincoln, E. (1989) *Fourth Generation Evaluation*, London: Sage.

Hammersley, M. (1992) *What's Wrong with Ethnography?*, London: Routledge.

Hammersley, M., Gomm, R. and Foster, P. (2000) 'Case study and theory', in R. Gomm, M. Hammersley and P. Foster (eds) *Case Study Method*, 234–58, London: Sage.

Hanlon, P., Beck, S., Robertson, G., Henderson, M., McQuillan, R., Capewell, S. and Dorward, A. (1997) 'Coping with the inexorable rise in medical admissions: evaluating a radical reorganisation of acute medical care in a Scottish district general hospital', *Health Bulletin*, 55, 3: 176–84.

Hart, E. and Bond, M. (1995) *Action Research for Health and Social Care: a Guide to Practice*, Milton Keynes, Open University Press.

Jick, T. D. (1979) 'Mixing qualitative and quantitative methods: triangulation in action', *Administrative Science Quarterly*, 24: 602–11.

Lewin, K. (1946) 'Action research and minority problems', *Journal of Social Issues*, 2: 34–46.

Meyer, J. (1993) 'New paradigm research in practice: the trials and tribulations of action research', *Journal of Advanced Nursing*, 18: 1066–72.

——(1995) 'Lay participation in care in a hospital setting: an action research study', Ph.D. thesis, University of London.

——(2000) 'Using qualitative methods in health related action research', *British Medical Journal*, 320: 178–81.

Meyer, J. and Bridges, J. (1998) *An Action Research Study into the Organisation of Care for Older People in the Accident and Emergency Department*, London: City University.

Potter, C., Morgan, P. and Thompson, A. (1994) 'Continuous quality improvement in an acute hospital: a report of an action research project in three hospital departments', *International Journal of Health Care Quality Assurance*, 7, 1: 5–29

Reason, P. and Rowan, J. (eds) (1981) *Human Inquiry: A Sourcebook of New Paradigm research*, Chichester: Wiley.

Rolfe, G. (1998) *Expanding Nursing Knowledge: Understanding and Researching Your Own Practice*, Oxford: Butterworth Heinemann.

Sackett, D. L., Richardson, W. S., Rosenberg, W. and Haynes, R. B. (1997) *Evidence-Based Medicine: How to Practice and Teach EBM*, Edinburgh: Churchill Livingstone.

Schon, D. A. (1987) *The Reflective Practitioner*, London: Temple Smith.

Sharp K. (1998) 'The case for case studies in nursing research: the problem of generalization', *Journal of Advanced Nursing*, 27: 785–9.

Simons, H. (1981) 'Process evaluation in schools', in C. Lacey and D. Lawton (eds) *Issues in Evaluation and Accountability*, London: Methuen.

Somekh, B. (1994) 'Inhabiting each other's castles: towards knowledge and mutual growth through collaboration', *Educational Action Research*, 2, 3: 357–81.

Stacey, J. (1988) 'Can there be a feminist ethnography?', *Women's Study International Forum*, 11, 1: 21–7.

Stringer, E. T. (1996) *Action Research: A Handbook for Practitioners*, London: Sage.

Susman, G. I. and Evered, R. D. (1978) 'An assessment of the scientific merits of action research', *Administrative Science Quarterly*, 23: 582–603.

Titchen, A. (2000) 'Professional craft knowledge in patient-centred nursing and the facilitation of its development', D.Phil. thesis, University of Oxford, Kidlington: Ashdale Press.

Walshe, K., Ham, C. and Appleby, J. (1995) 'Given in evidence', *Health Service Journal*, 29 June: 28–9.

Yin, R. K. (1994) *Case Study Research: Design and Methods*, 2nd edn, London: Sage.

Chapter 12

Synthesising research evidence

Nicholas Mays, Emilie Roberts and Jennie Popay

Introduction

This chapter discusses the synthesis of evidence in the field of delivery and organisation of health services. It aims to answer two questions:

- What are the particular challenges that reviewers investigating organisation and delivery of health services are likely to face?
- Given the wide range of disciplines and methods to be found in organisational research (both quantitative and qualitative), how can evidence from such studies be identified, selected and synthesised with confidence?

There is a large literature on methods to synthesise research evidence from studies that employ experimental designs, particularly randomised controlled trials of clinical interventions and drugs, and a reasonable degree of consensus as to how such syntheses should be undertaken. By contrast, there has been much less discussion, and still less agreement, on how to synthesise the evidence generated from other methods of research. This chapter focuses on the issues encountered in synthesising mainly non-experimental evidence, including qualitative data. It briefly covers the stages of such a review from defining the research question, through scoping the study, searching the literature, selecting relevant studies for inclusion, extracting data, assessing the quality of evidence in studies, to the analysis, presentation and interpretation of the findings.

The chapter concludes with a discussion of the problems likely to arise when reviewing service organisation and delivery. Organisations tend to be complex (being embedded within a wider health system and culture) and organisational behaviour is frequently not susceptible to experimental study. In addition, reviews in this area are often concerned with descriptive studies rather than comparisons of different interventions.

Definition and theoretical basis

The term 'systematic review' has been deliberately avoided, since this term is associated in some people's minds in the health field exclusively with reviews of randomised trials, in which data from different studies are pooled to calculate the overall effect of a particular treatment or pharmaceutical on health outcomes (Chalmers and Altman 1995). Combining data from different studies in reviews of non-experimental evidence will always be more problematic and involve non-statistical techniques.

This is not to say that reviews covering largely non-experimental quantitative and qualitative sources of data should be synonymous with what Mulrow (1987) termed 'traditional reviews' in contrast to systematic reviews, i.e. reviews which were subjective, lacked comprehensiveness, followed implicit procedures and were near-impossible to reproduce. Indeed, the approach to research synthesis described in this chapter has much in common with Mulrow's conception of a systematic review. Greenhalgh (1997) defines such a review as, 'an overview of primary studies which contains an explicit statement of objectives, materials and methods and has been conducted according to explicit and reproducible methodology'. As far as possible, this focus on comprehensiveness, explicitness about methods and reproducibility should also be the goal of researchers synthesising evidence from service delivery and organisational research, in order to limit bias and make conclusions more reliable. However, it is advisable for the researcher to be aware from the outset that there are far fewer hard-and-fast rules when synthesising findings from a range of different study designs, generating different sorts of data and driven by different theoretical and epistemological orientations. Formality and explicitness are desirable, but they have to be allied constantly to judgement, as this chapter will demonstrate.

Unlike the other research methods and disciplinary approaches discussed in the rest of this book, research syntheses or reviews are not necessarily the preserve of any one epistemological, theoretical or disciplinary perspective. For example, it may be possible to review research evidence from a particular theoretical perspective, but frequently the reviewer will wish to define the scope of the review in terms of a topic or subject area. In the latter case, the review process has to be capable of dealing with issues of generalisability, reliability and validity across different research traditions. There may well be occasions when theory and methods are incompatible between different pieces of research, and a simple cumulation of findings is not possible. On the other hand, the findings from studies of the same phenomenon carried out from different epistemological traditions can have the potential to improve understanding, even if the findings appear contradictory. The tension between perspectives can itself be enlightening.

The underlying assumption of research synthesis is that worthwhile insights, which cannot be obtained from simply reading the same set of studies sequentially, can be gained from simultaneously considering the accumulation of evidence from more than one study. This should not be taken to mean that research syntheses are necessarily a more accurate reflection of the true state of affairs than any one study, but simply that they afford opportunities for comparison and cumulation which are not possible with a single study, however robust.

Uses of research syntheses

Reviews of existing research are undertaken in the field of service delivery and organisation for the same broad reasons as in other fields. Research syntheses can be helpful in informing the decision making of policy makers, managers, practitioners and users of health services. These audiences value overviews which succinctly bring together a potentially large and often scattered body of research in a manageable way for quick absorption. Literature reviews are also an essential first step in the process of deciding whether any new research is required on an issue, by exposing the main gaps in knowledge, identifying the principal areas of dispute and uncertainty and, thereby, ensuring that any new research adds and connects to previous work rather than duplicates it, or fails to add meaningfully to it. Reviews can be pursued to answer specific questions which individual studies cannot shed light on. For example, if the bulk of the research in an area consists of case studies, it may be useful to attempt to synthesise their findings. Reviews can further help identify why different studies produce seemingly conflicting findings and draw out the hidden links between them.

Reviews can have other functions too. They can be useful in helping to choose between competing policy alternatives – for example, different models of community-based rehabilitation services, or different ways of providing support to informal carers. They can be useful in helping to shape the implementation of a course of action already determined (e.g. to identify the best way to provide a telephone health advice line by comparing the findings of a number of evaluations). They can also be used to identify a sub-set of settings and related findings, which relate most closely to the particular circumstances relevant to the reviewer.

How to undertake a research synthesis

'Cookbooks' and standards

There are many elements in common between reviews of randomised trials and of research using a broader range of study designs, particularly the importance of being explicit about the assumptions made and methods chosen. However, standards and methods developed for the former have to be used judiciously, not slavishly, for the latter. Nonetheless, it is useful to begin planning the review by reading one of the short published checklists for evaluating the quality of systematic reviews (Oxman 1995; Greenhalgh 1997; Khan *et al.* 2001). They encourage reviewers to prepare a formal review protocol containing the problem specification and the methods to be followed during the stages of formulating the review questions, search strategy, study selection (criteria and procedures), study quality assessment (checklists and procedures), data extraction and synthesis of extracted evidence. Preparing a written protocol, including a project timetable, is a helpful discipline as long as some flexibility is built into the subsequent review process, since it may be necessary to handle the stages more iteratively than some guidance would indicate. Another checklist worth consulting is Light and Pillemer's (1984), a modified version of which is summarised in Box 12.1, with additional questions from the current authors. This checklist has the advantage of having been framed to apply to both

---

Box 12.1 Checklist for undertaking and evaluating reviews of studies that compare two or more interventions

1 What is the precise purpose of the review? Are the review procedures related to that purpose?
2 Were the search methods used to find evidence relevant to the review clearly stated?
3 Was the search for evidence reasonably comprehensive?
4 Is there any evidence that steps were taken to minimise publication and other sources of bias in searching for evidence?
5 If inclusion/exclusion criteria were used, how were studies selected for inclusion? Are the implications of these criteria clear?
6 Were explicit criteria used for assessing the quality (freedom from bias) of the studies reviewed? Were these assessments used consistently to judge the weight to be given to the evidence from different studies? (e.g. have the findings [outcomes] from different studies been related to the type of research design?).
7 Have intervention groups been examined to see if they are similar in fact as well as in name?
8 Have comparison groups in different studies been examined for similarities and differences?
9 Is it easy to see the distribution of study outcomes?
10 Have the findings been related to the different features of programmes, participants and settings?

11 Is the unit of analysis (e.g. patient, ward, hospital, general practice) sufficiently similar across studies for meaningful comparisons to be made?

12 Were the findings of relevant studies combined appropriately where this was possible?

13 Were the conclusions of the review supported clearly by the evidence and analysis presented in the report?

14 Is there any guidance given on future research?

(*Note*: Questions 2, 3, 6, 12 and 13 have been added by the current authors; others have been slightly modified)

(Light and Pillemer 1984. Reprinted by permission of the publisher from *Summing Up: The Science of Reviewing Research*, by R. J. Light and D.B. Pillemer, Cambridge MA: Harvard University Press, copyright © 1984 by the President and Fellows of Harvard College.)

experimental and non-experimental evidence and to reviews in the social sciences, including those involving policy research, though it is limited to studies that evaluate interventions. It highlights the main decision-points encountered while undertaking a review but, unlike a 'cookbook', it does not attempt to resolve each one, since the solutions will depend on the topic under study, the nature of the evidence available, and the proportion of identified studies deemed acceptable for inclusion in the review.

Support and resourcing

Establishing a multidisciplinary advisory panel or steering group may be a wise precaution at the outset. Expertise in the relevant field will be particularly helpful in determining the likely timescale and staffing requirements for the review, since one of the most challenging tasks in synthesis in the current field is identifying in advance where the literature is likely to be located and how much useful material there is likely to be from different disciplines, sources and so on. Service delivery reviews can be surprisingly time-consuming, particularly when they involve identifying and synthesising different theoretical literatures. 'Expertise' should not be seen exclusively in academic and research terms: it can include the involvement of end-users of reviews, who may be managers, patients or advocates for particular client groups.

Information specialists and research librarians have expertise in constructing effective search strategies which researchers should make use of. Do not underestimate the costs involved in undertaking comprehensive searching for reviews. Apart from the researchers' own time and that of any supporting librarian or information scientist, the direct costs associated with searching, such as online access to electronic databases, purchase of CD-ROMs, inter-library loans and so on, can vary considerably. If the search strategy locates a large number of 'hits', then apparently trivial search-and-retrieval costs per item will mount up, before one even considers the cost of photocopying complete articles so that they can be read for potential inclusion in the review. It is sobering to note, as an example, that Lambert and Arblaster (2000) considered 56,000 abstracts for their review of factors associated with older people's admission to hospital.

Defining the research question

As in all research, this is a crucial step in undertaking any review. Questions can be either hypothesis-testing or exploratory (Light and Pillemer 1984). They can either seek to identify the 'average' effect of an intervention or the interaction, setting by setting and group by group, between an intervention and its effects, or expose the processes that shape the implementation of an intervention. In many cases of service delivery and organisational research, even where the aim is ostensibly to evaluate effectiveness, 'average' effects alone are unlikely to be very revealing guides to action for policy makers, and context-specific or sub-group questions will have to be pursued as well. This is key to good reviews in this field. Questions such as 'Which form of the organisational intervention or device, delivered by whom, is likely to be most effective for which client group in which settings and at what costs?' are likely to be the most pressing to answer, since most social interventions work better in some contexts than others and it is important to understand why, ahead of framing policy advice (Pawson and Tilley 1997).

At this stage, it is worth paying careful attention to definitions. Though these may change in light of the experience gained in undertaking the review, it is worth trying explicitly to define the subject matter of the review at the outset (hence the relevance of writing a review protocol), since it will become apparent as the literature is read that there are no consistent definitions in use in the field of service delivery and organisational research (Parker *et al.* 2000). For example, terms such as 'outpatient clinic', 'ambulatory care centre', 'polyclinic', 'primary care centre', 'health centre', 'patient-centred care', and so on may be used in different studies to define the same thing or something quite different in terms of ethos, clinical goals, staffing, range of services delivered and position relative to other parts of the health system. This is particularly likely when dealing with studies from more than one country, which is almost inevitable if the review is to be comprehensive.

Scoping to define the study domain and literature search strategy

Scoping and the early stages of searching the literature are frequently combined processes in service delivery and organisational reviews (hence the need to build some flexibility into the review protocol). Scoping studies aim to map *rapidly* the key concepts underpinning a research area and the main sources and types of evidence available, and can be undertaken as stand-alone projects in their own right, especially where an area is complex or has not been reviewed comprehensively before. Scoping is undertaken because it can be difficult to visualise the extent and distribution of the literature on a particular topic sufficiently well in advance to determine the limits of the domain of enquiry and plan the review in detail. Reviews often require the drawing of a 'map' of the literature informed by early searching and contact with subject area experts to identify broadly which parts, and how much, of the literature is likely to be relevant and can practicably be handled. The map is likely to be multi-layered (like a geological map), since researchers from different social sciences and with differing theoretical orientations can be expected to have studied the same phenomenon in different ways. This is rarely the case in undertaking systematic reviews of randomised trials of simple interventions, but should be expected in organisational and managerial research.

As well as offering opportunities for developing a deeper understanding of a single issue from more than one perspective, certain theoretical approaches may produce insights that are not commensurate with one another. Although this may not always be apparent before the stages of data extraction, analysis and synthesis have been completed, in some cases it is certain. For example, in Chapter 2 of this volume, functionalist organisational studies, which are designed to improve existing managerial performance, are compared with neo-Marxist studies, which are avowedly anti-managerialist and designed to lead to radically different forms of organisation of a type previously unknown under capitalist arrangements. The neo-Marxist studies can provide insights into how capitalist organisations operate which can be used in a less radical way to improve existing organisations, but the reviewer has to recognise that they were undertaken for an entirely different purpose.

Tensions and contrasts in the narrative synthesis are most likely to have to be handled when there are fundamental epistemological and value differences between researchers. In these situations, the work of rival traditions can be presented in separate sections of the narrative report for comparison, or an *explicit* decision can be taken to exclude a particular theoretical orientation from the scope of the review.

Synthesising the findings of extreme relativist research with other forms of either qualitative or quantitative investigation raises the further question of whether it is legitimate for a reviewer to use the findings of a study in a manner which the author would reject on epistemological grounds. Since the anti-realist position from which such research is conducted denies that there is any such thing as a social reality independent of the research process and any external means of judging the quality of a piece of research, then the idea of the cumulation of findings from different studies inherent in a review is meaningless from this perspective, as is the idea that research can provide any unequivocal insights for action (Murphy *et al.* 1998) (see Chapter 3 in this volume for further discussion of this issue). On the other hand, such studies usually present 'findings' and it is hard to see why reviewers should not be free to use these systematically to enhance their understanding, irrespective of the extreme relativist position adopted by the original authors. As a precaution, it might be wise to record the perspective from which the study was undertaken when extracting the data.

Sometimes the nature of the review question or topic will help in reducing the amount of theoretical dissonance. Thus, if the focus is less on the health care organisation as a whole and, for example, more on the contribution of different types of teams within it, the relevant research is more likely to come from occupational psychology rather than sociology. As has been seen in Chapter 5, the dominant paradigm in occupational psychology is positivist, adopted from the natural sciences. This is not the case in organisational sociology, where 'paradigm wars' are more common, thereby hindering straightforward quality assessment and synthesis of studies.

Searching

Given the multi-layered nature of the literature in many areas, and the difficulty of establishing a simple definition of scope, experience points to the need to start searches broadly, from multiple sources, and gradually increase the degree of focus as the review team becomes more familiar with the subject matter. Guides to systematic reviewing strongly advise that the search strategy be specified in advance in order to minimise reviewer bias. In principle, this is good advice, but rarely seems to correspond with the reality of searching on the sorts of topics likely to be encountered in the current field. On balance, it is more important to be flexible, but to document the process, including its twists and turns (and even blind alleys), so that others could potentially repeat it at a later date as new knowledge accumulates.

It is generally not advisable to rely on the keyword indexing available on the intervention or phenomenon of interest, when using bibliographic databases, since many electronic search engines were designed with clinical rather than organisational and managerial interests in mind. Frequently studies are not categorised in ways that help service delivery and organisational reviewers. Hand searching of journals and other sources that appear to be most productive from the results of prior searches is usually recommended but, given the wide range of journals in clinical and social science disciplines which may be relevant, working through the reference lists of papers and books which have already been identified can be more productive. Consulting subject area 'experts' at intervals during the search process can be very helpful, especially when it comes to identifying 'grey' literature (i.e. working papers, unpublished consultancy reports, etc.), work in progress and research published in unusual places. Subject area experts are particularly useful when a review is very broad (Le Grand *et al.* 1998).

When searching begins to produce very low yields in terms of studies previously unidentified, and the same references emerge again and again, it is probably time to stop and move on to determining which studies should be included in the final review. The goal is to try to be exhaustive within the original scope, but with reference to the time available for completing the review.

Selecting studies for inclusion

There are at least three main reasons why studies identified from the search may not be included in the eventual synthesis of evidence:

- the quality of the evidence contained in the study
- its relevance to the review
- the theoretical orientation of the study.

In most cases, the abstract of each paper will have to be read in order to assess its quality, relevance and theoretical orientation. Sometimes the assessment can only be finalised when the data have been extracted from each study. It is generally a good idea to use more than one assessor to define study inclusion based on the three criteria.

In most reviews, the search process and assessment of inclusion are designed to isolate studies that report findings, rather than theoretical or conceptual pieces. Thus a simple test of relevance for inclusion is to specify that each reference must relate to some form of *research, inquiry, investigation,* or *study*. This will eliminate a large amount of irrelevant commentary (e.g. from professional or 'trade' publications) at a reasonable cost in terms of missed evidence. Many of the references, particularly in the professional managerial literature, will turn out to contain neither conceptual nor empirical work, but comment and simple descriptions of local innovations. Some of this material will be well worth reading, particularly in the early orientation phase of the review (for example, it may identify how differently similar-seeming services are being implemented in practice, which is helpful in determining the relevance and comparability of different studies), but it is unlikely to find its way into the final data tables of the review.

Again, as in the searching stage, it is likely that reviewers will have to start broadly and gradually refine their inclusion criteria. There is no self-evidently 'correct' way to do this, so it is important that the reasoning is documented to enable future readers to assess the rigour of the review.

Assessing the quality of studies

Once a review extends its scope beyond randomised trials, the assessment of the *quality* of studies inevitably becomes more complex and more reliant on informed researcher judgement (Murphy *et al.* 1998). The challenge is to be able to identify 'good' research from whichever theoretical and methodological tradition it comes. This is a formidable undertaking because of the wide range of research methods and approaches available to social scientists which could be encountered in service delivery and organisational reviews. Given this breadth, quality criteria should be used primarily to assess the strength of the evidence from each study and, therefore, the weight each study's findings should be given in the synthesis and conclusions of the review, and only secondarily to eliminate the poorest-quality evidence from consideration in the first place. Ann Oakley has recently argued that

> the distinguishing mark of all 'good' research is the awareness and acknowledgement of error and that what flows from this is the necessity of establishing procedures which will minimise the effect such errors may have on what counts as knowledge.
>
> (Oakley 2000)

A number of classificatory schemes and assessment criteria have been devised for quantitative research, in general, designed to determine the degree to which findings are free from bias or error. One of the best known is the so-called 'hierarchy of evidence', a version of which is given in Box 12.2.

Box 12.2 An example of a 'hierarchy of evidence'

I Well designed randomised controlled trials

II Other types of trial:

II-1a Well designed controlled trials with pseudo-randomisation

II-1b Well designed controlled trials with no randomisation

Cohort studies:

II-2a Well-designed cohort (prospective study) with concurrent controls

II-2b Well-designed cohort (prospective study) with historical controls

II-2c Well-designed cohort (retrospective study) with concurrent controls
II-3 Well-designed case–control (retrospective) study
III Large differences from comparisons between times and/or places with and without intervention (in some circumstances these may be equivalent to level I or II)
IV Opinions of respected authorities based on clinical experience; descriptive studies; and reports of expert committees
(Centre for Reviews and Dissemination 1996)

Much of the assessment of the quality of quantitative health services research rests on this hierarchy, though to use it in practice requires detailed information on each study far beyond a simple description of its basic design. For example, a well designed observational study may well provide more useful evidence than a flawed randomised trial (Downs and Black 1998). Broadly speaking, the assessment is based on the degree to which a study design handles 'confounding' (i.e. its ability to rule out the possibility that observed, supposedly causal relationships, are due to the effects of unmeasured variables rather than the variables of interest) and thus assures the *internal* validity of the results. It does not consider the issue of *external* validity (i.e. generalisability) of the results.

There continues to be some debate about the criteria that should be used to assess the quality of quantitative studies, together with considerably more controversy over the relative weighting of each criterion. In addition, there is comparatively little evidence on the validity of the many instruments available even for assessing randomised trials (Moher *et al.* 1995). Given that little of the literature encountered in reviews in the service delivery field will be from randomised trials or susceptible to statistical meta-analysis, quality assessment of trials and meta-analysis are not discussed here.

A single 'hierarchy of evidence' is not appropriate for qualitative research, given the epistemological diversity of the field. However, there are general questions that can be asked to help judge 'validity' and 'reliability' in much qualitative research, in ways which overlap to some degree with the criteria used to appraise quantitative research, though they are not readily translated into simple checklists and scoring systems. A number of different schemes for assessing the quality of qualitative research have been developed. Three are summarised in Table 12.1.

They share many, but not all, criteria in common and can be used with care to develop assessment schemes for qualitative studies in service delivery reviews. Some writers have also successfully applied these schemes to quality appraisal of 'mixed' method studies which are common in the area of

Table 12.1 Three schemes for assessing the quality of qualitative health services research

Quality criterion or part of the research process	Mays and Pope 2000	Blaxter, on behalf of BSA Medical Sociology Group, 1996	Popay *et al.* 1998
Appropriateness of the methods used for the question(s) and subject matter	Would a different method have been more appropriate? Did the study require the use of qualitative methods? For example, if a causal hypothesis was being tested, was a qualitative approach really appropriate?	Are the methods of the research appropriate to the nature of the question being asked? i.e. does the research seek to understand processes or structures, or illuminate subjective experiences or meanings? Are the categories or groups being examined of a type which cannot be preselected, or the possible outcomes cannot be specified in advance? Could a quantitative approach have addressed the issue better? Does the sensitivity of the methods match the needs of the research questions? i.e. does the method accept the implications of an approach which respects the perceptions of those being studied?	Does the research, as reported, illuminate the subjective meaning, actions and context of those being researched? Popay *et al.* also regard the answer to this question as the first and main overall indicator of quality of a piece of qualitative health research, arguing that it should be answered before proceeding to answer the other subsidiary questions relating to the methodological soundness of the research.
Clarity of the research question	If not at the outset of the study, by the end of the research process was the research question clear?		

Table 12.1 Continued

Quality criterion or part of the research process	Mays and Pope 2000	Blaxter, on behalf of BSA Medical Sociology Group, 1996	Popay et al. 1998
Attention to context	Is the context/setting adequately described so that the reader can relate the findings to other settings?	Is the research clearly contextualised? i.e. is all the relevant information about the setting and subjects supplied?	Is there evidence of the adaptation and responsiveness of the research design to the circumstances and issues of real-life social settings met in the course of the study?
		Are the cases or variables which are being studied integrated in their social context, rather than being abstracted and decontextualised?	
Adequacy of sampling*	Did the sample include the full range of possible cases/settings so that statistical generalisations could be made (i.e. more than convenience sampling)?	Is there a clear account of the criteria used for the selection of subjects for study? Is the selection of cases or participants theoretically justified?	Does the sample produce the type of knowledge necessary to understand the structures and processes within which the individuals or situations are located?
	If appropriate, were efforts made to obtain data that might contradict or modify the analysis by extending the sample (e.g. including a different type of area)?		What claims are made for the generalisability of the findings to either bodies of knowledge or to other populations or groups?
Thoroughness of data collection*	Was the data collection process systematic?	Is there a clear account of the data collection methods?	
	Was an 'audit trail' provided, such that someone else could repeat each stage?	Are the limitations of any structured interview methods considered?	

Table 12.1 Continued

Quality criterion or part of the research process	Mays and Pope 2000	Blaxter, on behalf of BSA Medical Sociology Group, 1996	Popay et al. 1998
		If more than one worker was involved, has comparability been considered?	
		Was the data collection and record keeping systematic? Is the evidence available for independent examination?	
Rigour of data analysis*	Was the data analysis process systematic?	Is there a clear account of the data analysis?	How does the research move from a description of the data, through quotation or examples, to an analysis and interpretation of the meaning and significance of the research?
	Was an 'audit trail' provided, such that someone else could repeat each stage?	Is reference made to accepted procedures for analysis?	How are different sources of knowledge about the same issue compared and contrasted?
	How well did the analysis succeed in incorporating all the observations?	How systematic is the analysis?	
		Were full records or transcripts of conversations or summaries used if appropriate?	
	Was there unexplained variation?	Is there adequate discussion of how themes, concepts and categories were derived from the data?	
	To what extent did the analysis develop concepts and categories capable of explaining key processes or respondents' accounts or observations?	Are negative data presented? Has there been any search for cases which might refute the conclusions?	
	Was it possible to follow the iteration between data and the explanations for the data (theory)?	Have measures been taken to test the validity of findings (e.g. respondent validation, triangulation)?	
	Did the researcher seek disconfirming cases?	Has reliability been considered, ideally by independent repetition?	

Table 12.1 Continued

Quality criterion or part of the research process	Mays and Pope 2000	Blaxter, on behalf of BSA Medical Sociology Group, 1996	Popay et al. 1998
Reflexivity of the account	Was the researcher able to set aside his/her research preconceptions? Did the researcher self-consciously assess the likely impact of the methods used on the data obtained?	Is the author's own position clearly stated? Has the researcher examined his/her own role, possible bias and influence on the research? Is there adequate discussion of the evidence for and against the researcher's arguments?	Are subjective perceptions and experiences, including those of the researcher, treated as knowledge in their own right?
Adequacy of presentation of findings	Were sufficient data included in the report of the study to allow readers to assess whether analytical criteria (see above) had been met?	Are the data presented systematically? Do the conclusions follow from the data? Is sufficient original evidence presented to satisfy the reader of the relationship between the evidence and the conclusions? Are quotations, etc. identified in such a way that the reader can judge the range of evidence being used?	Is the description detailed enough to allow the researcher or reader to interpret the meaning and context of what is being researched?

Table 12.1 Continued

Quality criterion or part of the research process	Mays and Pope 2000	Blaxter, on behalf of BSA Medical Sociology Group, 1996	Popay et al. 1998
Attention to ethical issues		Have ethical issues been adequately considered? i.e. is the issue of confidentiality adequately dealt with; have the consequences of the research been considered (e.g. in terms of relationships with subjects, raised expectations, changed behaviour, etc.)?	
		Has the relationship between fieldworkers and subjects been considered and is there evidence that the research was presented and explained to its subjects?	
Worth/relevance of the research overall	Was this piece of research worth doing at all?	Is the connection to an existing body of knowledge or theory clear?	Does the research, as reported, illuminate the subjective meaning, actions and context of those being researched?
	Has it contributed usefully to knowledge?	Are the results credible and appropriate? i.e. do they address the research question; are they plausible and coherent; are they important, either theoretically or practically, or trivial?	How relevant is the research to policy and/or practice?

Note: * It is recognised that the separation between 'sampling', 'data collection', 'data analysis', interpretation and 'presentation of findings' is rarely clear, nor necessarily desirable in qualitative studies.

service delivery and organisation – for example, in systematic reviews of process evaluations of health promotion interventions (Harden *et al.* 1999). However, they all suffer from the drawback that they do not spell out in detail *how* each criterion should be applied: in particular, how to discern whether or not a sufficient standard has been reached with respect to any of the quality criteria. Admittedly, similar difficulties have been reported with respect to algorithms for assessing the quality of quantitative studies (Parker *et al.* 2000).

Much rests on the judgement of the reviewer. Two main criteria stand out from the different approaches (see Table 12.1) – validity and relevance – both of which are also important for assessing quantitative research (Hammersley 1990). The difference between the assessment of qualitative or 'mixed'-method research and studies aimed at measuring quantitative outcomes, lies not in the fundamental criteria so much as how they are operationalised and used. For example, a quantitative study might be assessed for validity in terms of the efforts made by the researchers to falsify a prior hypothesis. The equivalent for a qualitative study would be an assessment of the lengths to which the researchers went in attempting to identify negative or 'deviant' cases and to build them into their explanation – that is, their attention to elements in the data, which appeared to contradict the emerging explanation of the phenomenon under study. However, it is important to note that the logic underlying the former is to use exceptions to *disprove* a hypothesis, whereas the latter approach analyses exceptions to *improve* the quality of the explanation (or 'theory') (Barbour 1999).

Finally, there are likely to be specific quality criteria relating to studies of service delivery and organisation which are relatively more important in this field than elsewhere, irrespective of their designs. For example, a study which did not define unequivocally and in detail what was meant by terms such as 'hospital-at-home' or 'intermediate care' would be automatically of low quality since it would be impossible to compare with other studies on the same broad topic.

Another salient quality issue in service delivery studies relates to the unit of data collection and analysis used. Health services researchers have only relatively recently become fully sensitive to the importance of elucidating the different levels at which different types of interventions have their effect (see Chapter 4). Typically, service delivery and organisational changes and specific interventions are delivered to institutional or geographic sub-units, or to groups of staff or patients. For example, a new form of peer review in general practice is likely to be focused on groups of GPs and will have its effect at the group level, so that data either on GPs' behaviour or on patient outcomes must be grouped accordingly (i.e. the unit of analysis is the groups of doctors) (Ukoumunne *et al.* 1999; Wood and Freemantle 1999). As a consequence, different considerations may enter into quality assessments depending on the subject matter of the review in question. Thus quality assessment of studies for reviews in the current field should be regarded as analogous to the acceptance decisions of a journal editor rather than the scores produced by a straightforward checklist. The most important point is to have quality criteria, which are used consistently either for inclusion/exclusion decisions, and/or during the synthesis and analysis of findings, which are explicit and reproducible as far as possible.

Analysis and synthesis of findings

Having scoped, searched and decided how to appraise the evidence and what to include, the next stage is to synthesise the data in a way that is accessible and convincing. Synthesising data from a set of studies, which may span many countries, over many years, and incorporate a variety of different methods and theoretical perspectives, is probably the single most challenging task facing the reviewer.

There are three basic approaches to the synthesis of evidence in reviews: *narrative, tabular* and *statistical*. The balance between these approaches will depend on the set of studies available for the review. Most reviews in the service delivery and organisation field will predominantly use both narrative and tabular approaches. Much of the analysis included in reviews of service delivery and organisation can reasonably be described as involving some elements of synthesis. Synthesising findings from 'mixed'-method studies is likely to be aimed at identifying dominant and/or recurrent themes in the studies, or common contextual factors which impinge on the implementation of initiatives. Systematic exploration of why study results *differ* (as they are likely to do), and of the relationship between the potentially contrasting insights from qualitative and quantitative enquiries, will be more illuminating in this field than identifying average effects. Seemingly unpatterned findings in different directions from quantitative studies may be shown to have underlying consistency when study design, details of the settings, staff types, patient characteristics, programme details, and year or season of data collection, as well as qualitative features of the setting such as the nature of the organisational culture, are taken into account.

Qualitative information may be crucial in identifying factors that may enable or impede the implementation of a policy or intervention (e.g. aspects of the culture of a local health system), thereby helping explain seemingly anomalous findings between quantitative studies, and producing a more subtle interpretation of the evidence (Barbour 1999). It can also be useful in capturing participants' subjective evaluations of the implementation and outcomes of an organisational change. In addition, qualitative findings can be used to generate theories to be tested in future quantitative research as well as identifying the relevant variables for study.

Synthesis of findings across diverse study designs is far from simple and will always take a narrative form, in the sense of being reported in textual rather than numerical terms. However, this does not mean that formalised systematic approaches are not possible. Three such narrative approaches to synthesis of findings across diverse study designs can be identified, in addition to simple tabular summaries, and they may be used in tandem rather than being mutually exclusive: *theory-led*, *analytical* and *triangulation*.

Within qualitative (and arguably all) research, theory has a pivotal role in informing the interpretation of data. The extent to which researchers have sought to link their work to wider theoretical frames is a key aspect of the schemes developed for assessing the quality of qualitative research as discussed above. However, theory may also provide a valuable framework within which to explore the relationship between findings from different studies, including findings within and across qualitative and quantitative studies (Williams *et al.* 1999). In their recent review of peer-led approaches to health promotion aimed at young people, for example, Harden and colleagues (Box 12.3) considered the relationship between findings from diverse studies in the context of theories relating to aspects of control and autonomy experienced by young people in their personal lives.

Box 12.3 Synthesis of findings from research using mixed methods

Review question

'What is the effectiveness and appropriateness of peer-delivered health promotion for young people?'

Outcome evaluations were used to address questions of effectiveness, and process evaluations were used to address the questions of appropriateness. Appropriateness included examining which factors promote or impede the implementation of peer-delivered health promotion initiatives. Whether it is more appropriate or effective than traditional approaches was a 'sub-question'. A guiding factor in the decision to include process evaluations was a response to policy and practitioner needs for information on process as well as outcome.

Population

Young people aged eleven to twenty-four years old.

Interventions

Peer-delivered health promotion initiatives across a range of health topics including drugs, smoking, safe sex and diet. Interventions could consist of skill development, awareness raising or other approaches, as long as they were provided to young people by their peers. Studies could compare peer-delivered interventions to those delivered by adults or to groups receiving no intervention.

Outcomes

A range of outcomes including health-related behaviours, attitudes, intentions and knowledge.

Processes

Acceptability and accessibility of the intervention, factors influencing the implementation of the intervention, collaborations and partnerships, and delivery of the intervention.

Study designs

Effectiveness: RCTs/non-randomised trials/cohort studies using quantitative outcomes.

Process evaluation: Studies using both quantitative and qualitative methods.

Synthesis of results from effectiveness studies

There were twelve effectiveness studies which were judged to be sound. Non-quantitative synthesis showed that more studies demonstrated peer-delivered health promotion to be effective than ineffective. However, it was not possible to identify specific characteristics of an effective model of peer-delivered health promotion.

Synthesis of results from process evaluation studies

There were fifteen process evaluations, of which two were embedded within effectiveness studies. The process evaluations included a range of designs, and only two met all the quality criteria identified. Synthesis of findings identified the following factors/processes that may influence the outcome of peer-led interventions.

- *Acceptability*: young people are more likely to express a preference for peer-led sessions in comparison to teacher-led sessions, and to perceive peer leaders as credible sources of information.
- *Factors influencing implementation*: many factors were identified; conflict between the philosophy of peer education as a non-traditional educational strategy and its implementation in more traditional school settings was particularly common.
- *Training and personal development of peer leaders*: ongoing support for peer educators was identified as a high priority.
- *Accessibility*: young people acting as peer educators might be most comfortable working with their friends, and even in this context may feel that the

advice and/or information they were to transmit would be seen as 'interfering'.

- *Recruitment of peer leaders*: peer leaders were more likely to be female; once recruited, it was more difficult to retain male peer leaders.
- *Working in partnership with young people*: the potential for conflict between adult coordinators of interventions and the peer leaders they were supporting was identified; in particular, adults involved could find it difficult to deal with the increasing confidence of peer leaders and their emerging ideas, wants and needs.

(Harden *et al.* 1999)

A second approach could be described as analytical. The idea of conducting analytical syntheses of findings across qualitative research studies is not new. For example, when Glaser and Strauss (1967) developed their now well established method of 'grounded theory', they argued for comparisons between sites and cases in order to increase the generality of a finding or explanation in qualitative research. Some of the techniques developed to aid the synthesis of qualitative data across sites/cases assume that the data have been collected within the context of a single study. This is the case with the meta-matrices proposed by Miles and Huberman (1994) for instance. Other approaches, such as the methods for meta-ethnography proposed by Noblit and Hare (1988), are designed to be used across different studies. As with statistical meta-analysis there is a need for careful assessment of the comparability of the data to be synthesised, and access to raw data – in the form of transcripts, for example – may be needed. However, in theory at least, these analytical techniques could be applied to synthesis of findings from qualitative studies and to the integration of qualitative and quantitative findings.

Third, and closely related to the above, the literature on triangulation (see Chapter 1) within the social sciences is relevant to the synthesis of findings from diverse study designs within the context of a systematic review. This is a widely used approach to exploring the validity of, and relationship between, research findings through the systematic comparison of data collected from different perspectives. Although it usually involves comparisons of qualitative and quantitative data collected during the same study, this approach can be used with data from different studies.

There are, inevitably, theoretical objections to *any* attempt to combine findings from qualitative and quantitative studies. Ackroyd and Hughes (1992), for example, question the epistemological validity of the triangulation of qualitative and quantitative data, arguing that there are no 'criteria upon which all agree and which can be used to decide between alternative theories, methods and inconsistencies in findings'. In contrast, Mason (1994) makes a strong case for the synthesis of different types of data, arguing that the key question is 'What are all the components necessary for generating a viable and convincing explanation and how do we get to that point?' (see Chapter 3).

Presentation of findings

The 'synthesis' and 'presentation' of findings are best thought of as parts of the same process, especially when there are, say, thirty or more studies in the review. It will not be possible to begin to reach a synthesis of the studies in this situation until an approach to summarising and presenting their findings has been developed. Once the studies have been summarised, it is possible to use the more ambitious techniques of narrative synthesis discussed above (theory-led, analysis-led and triangulation-based). The best guidance on the presentation of findings is to look at the tables and figures in published reviews in relevant fields.

Most reviews will require a detailed descriptive table or tables covering aspects of each study, such as: authors, year, detail of the intervention/initiative, nature of the comparator (if relevant), theoretical basis, design, quality assessment (relevant to the theoretical and design features of the study), outcomes (and costs, if relevant) measured, setting/context, population/participants (e.g. of areas, institutions, departments, clinicians, patients, etc.), main findings, implications for policy or practice, and general comments. Normally, the methods and results from studies have to be presented in separate tables, otherwise the tables become unwieldy. Almost invariably, specific reviews will require particular dimensions of studies to be summarised which are not relevant in other circumstances. Depending on the topic and the nature of the research evidence, separate tables may be needed on qualitative and quantitative studies, or the qualitative evidence may be used to help explain the quantitative findings. Economic data may be presented separately on occasion.

The tables ensure that the review is potentially reproducible and can be subjected easily to subsequent scrutiny. However, bulky tables listing methods and data from individual studies are generally unreadable to anyone simply wanting to learn the answer to the research question posed by the review. The reviewer has to go beyond this form of tabular presentation to produce a tabular synthesis, summarising the key findings in an accessible way.

The final report from the review is thus likely to include a series of summary tables which it is worth sketching out at the beginning of the synthesis stage in addition to the tables of individual studies. Most reports start with a table describing the designs and 'quality' of the studies to be reviewed, perhaps followed by a table or figure describing the distribution of studies in terms of their specific focus (e.g. detailed interventions) or the specific comparisons they make, or the outcomes included (Box 12.4).

Box 12.4 The distribution of studies of the effect of different interventions on the use of hospital emergency services

Primary care interventions studied	Frequency with which intervention has been studied
Better access for a population with lower than average income/poor availability of low-cost primary care	* * * * * * *
'Comprehensive' primary care	* * * * * *
Emergency on-call cover	* * * * *
Primary care service for children	* * *
Capitation payment or salary	* * *
Multidisciplinary team	* *
Specialist doctors	* *
Restrictions on hospital access	* *
Nurse-practitioners	* *
Home visits	* *
Emergency treatment room	*
Telephone advice	*
Advocacy/interpreting	*

Source: Roberts and Mays 1998

In the presentation of findings from comparative quantitative studies, a range of techniques should be considered. These include frequency distributions of effect sizes, funnel displays of outcomes such as effect sizes against aspects of study quality such as sample size, or simple 'voting' methods (e.g. counting up the significantly 'negative', significantly 'positive' and equivocal or 'mixed' studies or outcomes). When using simple counts of studies, care is needed to ensure that the quality of studies has already been taken into account when selecting which studies to synthesise (Box 12.5), or factored into the presentation or discussion of the findings. In addition, it is important to be as concerned with explaining why some studies differ from the rest, as with identifying the overall 'direction' of the findings.

In the presentation of results from the synthesis of studies involving qualitative or 'mixed' methods, summary tables might include descriptions of the key points or dominant themes identified in the synthesis (Box 12.3).

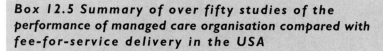

Box 12.5 Summary of over fifty studies of the performance of managed care organisation compared with fee-for-service delivery in the USA

(Steiner and Robinson 1998)

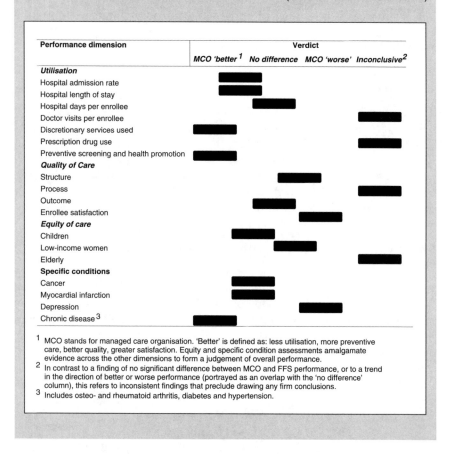

Performance dimension	Verdict			
	MCO 'better'[1]	No difference	MCO 'worse'	Inconclusive[2]
Utilisation				
Hospital admission rate	■			
Hospital length of stay	■			
Hospital days per enrollee		■		
Doctor visits per enrollee				■
Discretionary services used	■			
Prescription drug use				■
Preventive screening and health promotion	■			
Quality of Care				
Structure		■		
Process				■
Outcome		■		
Enrollee satisfaction			■	
Equity of care				
Children	■			
Low-income women		■		
Elderly				■
Specific conditions				
Cancer	■			
Myocardial infarction	■			
Depression			■	
Chronic disease[3]	■			

[1] MCO stands for managed care organisation. 'Better' is defined as: less utilisation, more preventive care, better quality, greater satisfaction. Equity and specific condition assessments amalgamate evidence across the other dimensions to form a judgement of overall performance.

[2] In contrast to a finding of no significant difference between MCO and FFS performance, or to a trend in the direction of better or worse performance (portrayed as an overlap with the 'no difference' column), this refers to inconsistent findings that preclude drawing any firm conclusions.

[3] Includes osteo- and rheumatoid arthritis, diabetes and hypertension.

Structure of a typical review report

Following the approach outlined in this chapter should lead to a review report which is structured broadly as follows:

- Summary
- Background
- Questions addressed by the review
- Review methods, including search strategy, data sources used, study quality assessment and any selection criteria used pre-synthesis stage, data extraction, data synthesis

- Details of included and excluded studies (can be as an appendix)
- Findings, including tabular presentation of findings (either thematic or quantitative) and a narrative synthesis (e.g. using theory-led, analytical or triangulation approaches)
- Discussion of the studies, including the interpretation of their findings, an assessment of the robustness of the results, explanations for any heterogeneity in results and implications for policy, practice and future research
- Conclusions.

Limitations

This chapter has already discussed some of the more obvious challenges that need to be faced in undertaking reviews in the current field, such as the greater reliance on explicit judgement (for example, of research quality) and the difficulty of comparing and aggregating the findings of studies undertaken from differing theoretical and methodological positions. However, there are other challenges when reviewing studies that compare the impact of different interventions or of different ways of implementing services.

Complexity of interventions and programmes of interest

In the field of service delivery and organisation, the subjects of review are frequently complex interventions or modifications to services, which may have multiple objectives and may have their effect at more than one level in the health system. Interventions may affect all or some of the structure, organisation, financing, payment, location, mode of delivery, identity of staff and other features of a service (Box 12.6).

> **Box 12.6 A theoretically informed narrative synthesis: the impact of organisational and managerial factors on the quality of care in health care organisations**
>
> Flood reviewed studies of the quality of care delivered in hospitals in terms of the impact of the following features on outcomes: physicians' training and experience; the training and experience of other staff; formal procedures and policies; the nature of the hospitals as 'workshops' (i.e. their equipment and infrastructure); and the hospitals' places in the local health system (e.g. the extent to which their actions were coordinated with those of other institutions).

While the review summarises a large body of primary research, its main purpose is to highlight the limitations of the available research in explaining the processes by which organisations affect the quality of care, and to identify key questions for future research using a more sophisticated model of the relationships between organisational structure, processes and outcomes than had generally been used in empirical research to date. As a result, the empirical research reviewed is placed in a theoretical context before it is summarised and interpreted. For example, research that focuses on the impact of the quality of the individual professionals in the health care organisation is framed in terms of 'agency theory', which deals with the incentives facing informed professionals acting on behalf of less well-informed patients.

(Flood 1994)

The importance of context for generalisability of findings

Initiatives relating to service delivery have their effects within, and are conditioned by, contexts and local and regional systems of care (Sheldon 2001). They are social programmes, not technological 'fixes' such as pharmaceuticals. The boundary between the particular programme and its context is not always easy to identify, and seemingly similar programmes can have different effects depending on where in the system of care they are located, what the local clinical culture is like, factors such as the degree of competition between providers, how they are managed, the level and quality of staff, and

Box 12.7 Are studies comparable? The impact of payment systems on the behaviour of primary care physicians

Although Gosden and colleagues did not consider studies in which an existing payment system was altered (e.g. by altering fee levels), focusing exclusively on studies which compared different systems of payment, they found very considerable heterogeneity in study settings, outcomes measured, reporting of findings and the interventions in question which made it difficult to compare studies. As a result, it was not possible to draw robust conclusions for use in a range of policy contexts.

> Had the study included other potentially influential features of the basic payment systems such as, in fee-for-service settings, who pays (patient, private insurer or government), how much they pay in relation to the full cost of delivering the service and whether the patient pays in advance and has to seek retrospective reimbursement, or is reimbursed directly (i.e. the physician claims the fee on behalf of the patient), the extent of comparability would have been further reduced.
>
> (Gosden *et al.* 2001)

so on. This is a more general formulation of the point about the complexity of subject matter discussed above (Box 12.7).

By contrast, chemically, a drug is identical wherever it is administered. Sources of variability in its effects relate to how it is administered, the dosage and patient characteristics rather than to changes in the entity itself. Thus the potential range of variation is generally less in drug trials, and the generalisability of individual studies is considerably greater as a result.

Another obvious factor affecting simple notions of generalisability of

Box 12.8 Identifying the relevant comparator: substituting improved access to primary care for use of the hospital Accident and Emergency department

In a review designed to assess the extent to which secondary/primary care substitution was possible in the field of first-contact, emergency care, Roberts and Mays noted that improving first contact, general practitioner care in the Accident and Emergency department (emergency room) of a hospital serving a deprived community was likely to have very different results compared with the status quo in different health systems, such as that of the USA compared with the UK. In the USA, the relevant status quo comparator in studies tended to comprise the prevailing low level of access to relatively few primary care physicians enjoyed by deprived populations. As a result, the reported effects of interventions tended to be very pronounced in terms of their impact on quality and timeliness of care and hospital admissions averted. In the UK, the impact of such interventions on hospital use and quality of care would be likely

to be far more modest, since most people, even in deprived populations, have reasonable access to a tolerable level of primary care
services.

(Roberts and Mays 1998)

findings relates to the relevance of the comparator used in the research,
which may vary from context to context (Box 12.8).

The importance of context for the relevance of findings

The selection of a particular drug or intervention by clinicians is frequently
shaped both by considerations of cost-effectiveness ('rational' considerations) and by cultural and historical factors (e.g. the traditionally greater
propensity of French physicians to use radiological techniques than British).
This is even more so in the case of the shape of the health care delivery
system. The range of options perceived as feasible at any one time is conditioned by deep-rooted political and cultural assumptions, and constrained

Box 12.9 The importance of context for relevance of findings: the impact of managed care on the cost and quality of health care

The aim of the review was to draw research-based conclusions, which
would be relevant to the National Health Service in the UK. Yet the
vast bulk of research on so-called 'managed care' was from the USA,
and compared capitated managed care organisations of different
types with fee-for-service medical practice under traditional third-
party payer indemnity insurance. While the use of capitation as one
element in 'managed care' was highly relevant to policy makers in
publicly financed health systems such as in the UK and New Zealand,
the comparison with fee-for-service under traditional private medical
insurance was not relevant.

In addition, there was almost no research directly related to the
effects of the micro techniques of managed care as opposed to
managed care organisations as a whole. Yet techniques such as utilisation review and physician profiling were the elements of managed
care most relevant for policy in publicly financed health systems such
as in the UK. As a result, the authors were forced to conclude:

> A thorough examination of this evidence has revealed a multitude of revealing and important findings but it does not suggest that they are directly applicable to the NHS. We believe that this is an important conclusion given the many claims made by managed care enthusiasts in the UK.
>
> (Robinson and Steiner 1998)

by the institutional history of the country in question (see Chapter 9). Thus the comparisons available within the empirical literature may not be politically practicable in the country that wishes to make use of the findings of the research (Box 12.9).

The timing of research may also affect its relevance in subtle ways, since health systems are dynamic, like medical technologies. For instance, the effect of a hospital-at-home scheme in reducing inpatient bed days is likely to be far greater in a period when hospital stays are longer than when stays have been reduced. Sometimes the reviewer needs up-to-date, 'softer' intelligence about the field to be able to interpret more formal research evidence correctly. For example, Robinson (2000) hypothesised that one of the reasons why US 'managed care' in all its many manifestations appeared to be relatively benign in its effects when the latest research evidence was synthesised at the end of the 1990s (Box 12.9), yet attracted such a high level of popular animosity at the same time, was because managed care organisations were changing so quickly that the research evidence almost inevitably related to forms which no longer existed by the time findings were published. In these cases, reviews may legitimately be limited in scope to studies from countries with broadly comparable health systems, or studies carried out in the recent past. This is particularly likely to be necessary if the aim of the review is 'summative' (i.e. it aims to reach a definitive conclusion) rather than exploratory. Of course, any geographic or temporal restrictions incorporated into the scope and search strategy should be clearly set out and justified.

Identifying relevant studies

In a review of the best place of care for older people after an acute illness, the authors noted that some outcomes (effects of service delivery interventions) can be interventions in their own right elsewhere in the local system (Parker *et al.* 2000). As a result, there may be evidence relevant to a review concerned with the best place of care for older people after acute hospital treatment, buried in the literature on long-term care and which may not have anything explicitly to do with aftercare following admission to an acute hospital.

Parker and colleagues also point to the difficulty in certain situations of distinguishing between *clinical* interventions and *locations* of care (the latter being relevant to service delivery reviews), since certain interventions may be more or less likely to be offered in different settings. There can also be inter-actions between the setting and the success of the type of care. For example, specialist care may be more effective in a specialist setting than the same care delivered in a generalist setting. This indicates the importance of framing the original review question carefully. High-level comparisons of 'hospital' versus 'community' versus 'home' care are unlikely to be enlightening in most cases, because they conceal rather than reveal the nature of the differ-ences in types of care assumed to be associated with each location. They are also unlikely to provide much of an indication in themselves as to why there might be differences in outcomes associated with different locations of care.

Unfortunately for reviewers of studies of service delivery, there is a consid-erable amount of health services research which is concerned with organisations, but which tends to treat them as a 'black box' (Chapter 1), so that it is not possible to determine *why* some studies show better or worse or different outcomes from others. In these studies, organisations are reduced to a handful of labels such as 'teaching hospital' or 'non-teaching hospital', with little attention paid to the processes taking place within hospitals in each type. From a service delivery perspective, such research would prove to be largely irrelevant unless it also reported the ways in which particular institutional arrangements affected the quality of service and patient outcomes. Robinson (2000) points out that most of the research on the costs and outcomes associ-ated with different forms of managed care in the USA is of this 'black box' type, thereby reducing its relevance outside the USA (Box 12.9).

To review or not?

The review of the literature on the best place of care for older people after acute illness, discussed above, concluded by raising the question of whether 'systematic review techniques' were useful at all in the area of service delivery and organisation (Parker *et al.* 2000). The authors were apparently disheartened by the complexity and uncertainty inherent in many of the issues that have been discussed in this chapter, and by the fact that many of the systematic review procedures developed for clinical interventions or drugs, which they had tried to mobilise, could not be used straightforwardly in management and organisation research. Yet their review was able to show that recent service developments in Britain were in precisely the areas where they had been able to conclude that evidence of effectiveness was weakest – hardly an inconsequential finding! Whatever the limitations of comprehen-sive reviews in service delivery and organisational fields, it is hard to see how good new research can be commissioned and undertaken without a thorough knowledge of what has already been accomplished. For this reason alone, good reviews will continue to be needed in these fields.

Further reading

Chalmers, I. and Altman, D. G. (eds) (1995) *Systematic reviews*, London: BMJ Books.

Khan, K. S., Ter Riet, G., Glanville, J., Sowden, A. J. and Kleijnen, J. (eds) for the NHS Centre for Reviews and Dissemination (2001) *Undertaking Systematic Reviews of Research on Effectiveness: CRD's Guidance for Carrying out or Commissioning Reviews*, 2nd edn, CRD Report no. 4, York: NHS Centre for Reviews and Dissemination, University of York.

 Light, R. J. and Pillemer, D. B. (1984) *Summing Up: The Science of Reviewing Research*, Cambridge MA: Harvard University Press.

Popay, J., Rogers, A. and Williams, G. (1998) 'Rationale and standards for the systematic review of qualitative literature in health services research', *Qualitative Health Research*, 8: 341–51.

References

Ackroyd, S. and Hughes, J. (1992) *Data Collection in Context*, London: Longman.

Barbour, R. (1999) 'The case for combining qualitative and quantitative approaches in health services research', *Journal of Health Services Research and Policy*, 4: 39–43.

Blaxter, M., on behalf of the BSA Medical Sociology Group (1996) 'Criteria for evaluation of qualitative research', *Medical Sociology News*, 22: 68–71.

Centre for Reviews and Dissemination (1996) *Undertaking Systematic Reviews of Research on Effectiveness*, CRD Report 4, York: NHS Centre for Reviews and Dissemination, University of York.

Chalmers, I. and Altman, D. G. (eds) (1995) *Systematic reviews*, London: BMJ Books.

Downs, S. H. and Black, N. A. (1998) 'The feasibility of creating a checklist for the assessment of the methodological quality both of randomised and non-randomised studies of health care interventions', *Journal of Epidemiology and Community Health*, 52: 377–84.

Flood, A. B. (1994) 'The impact of organizational and managerial factors on the quality of care in health care organizations', *Medical Care Review*, 51: 381–428.

Glaser, B. G. and Strauss, A. L. (1967) *The Discovery of Grounded Theory: Strategies for Qualitative Research*, Chicago: Aldine.

Gosden, T., Forland, F., Kristiansen, I. S., Sutton, M., Leese, B., Giuffrida, A., Sergison, M. and Pedersen, L. 'Impact of payment method on behaviour of primary care physicians: a systematic review', *Journal of Health Services Research and Policy*, 6: 44–55.

Greenhalgh, T. (1997) 'Papers that summarise other papers (systematic reviews and meta-analyses)', *British Medical Journal*, 315: 672–5.

Hammersley, M. (1990) *Reading Ethnographic Research*, New York: Longman.

Harden, A., Weston, R. and Oakley, A. (1999) *A Review of the Effectiveness and Appropriateness of Peer-delivered Health Promotion for Young People*, London: Social Science Research Unit, Institute of Education, University of London.

Khan, K. S., Ter Riet, G., Glanville, J., Sowden, A. J. and Kleijnen, J. (eds) for the NHS Centre for Reviews and Dissemination (2001) *Undertaking Systematic Reviews of Research on Effectiveness: CRD's Guidance for Carrying out or Commissioning Reviews*, 2nd edn, CRD Report no. 4, York: NHS Centre for Reviews and Dissemination, University of York.

Lambert, M. and Arblaster, L. (2000) 'Factors associated with acute use of hospital beds by older people: a systematic review of the literature', in Department of Health, *Shaping the Future NHS: Long Term Planning for Hospitals and Related Services*, consultation document on the findings of the National Beds Inquiry – supporting analysis, Annex G, London: Department of Health.

Le Grand, J., Mays, N. and Mulligan, J.-A. (eds) (1998) *Learning from the NHS Internal Market: A Review of the Evidence*, London: King's Fund.

Light, R. J. and Pillemer, D. B. (1984) *Summing Up: The Science of Reviewing Research*, Cambridge MA: Harvard University Press.

Mason, J. (1994) 'Linking qualitative and quantitative data analysis', in A. Bryman and R. G. Burgess (eds) *Analysing Qualitative Data*, 89–110, London: Routledge.

Mays, N. and Pope, C. (2000) 'Quality in qualitative health research', in C. Pope and N. Mays (eds) *Qualitative Research in Health Care*, 2nd edn, 89–101 London: BMJ Books.

Miles, M. B. and Huberman, A. M. (1994) *Qualitative Data Analysis: an Expanded Source Book*, 2nd edn, Thousand Oaks, CA: Sage.

Moher, D., Jadad, A. R., Nichol, G., Penman, M., Tugwell, P. and Walsh, S. (1995) 'Assessing the quality of randomised controlled trials: an annotated bibliography of scales and checklists', *Controlled Clinical Trials*, 16: 62–73.

Mulrow, C. D. (1987) 'The medical review article: state of the science', *Annals of Internal Medicine*, 106: 485–8.

Murphy, E., Dingwall, R., Greatbach, D., Parker, S. and Watson, P. (1998) 'Qualitative research methods in health technology assessment: a review of the literature', *Health Technology Assessment*, 2, 16: 1–276.

Noblit, G. W. and Hare, R. D. (1988) *Meta-ethnography: Synthesizing Qualitative Studies*, Newbury Park CA: Sage.

Oakley, A. (2000) *Experiments in Knowing: Gender and Method in Social Sciences*, Cambridge: Polity Press.

Oxman, A. D. (1995) 'Checklists for review articles', in I. Chalmers and D. G. Altman (eds) *Systematic Reviews*, 75–85, London: BMJ Books.

Parker, G., Bhakta, P., Katbamna, S., Lovett, C., Paisley, S., Parker, S., Phelps, K., Baker, R., Jagger, C., Lindesay, J., Shepherdson, B. and Wilson, A. (2000) 'Best place of care for older people after acute and during subacute illness: a systematic review', *Journal of Health Services Research and Policy*, 5, 176–89.

Pawson, R. and Tilley, N. (1997) *Realistic Evaluation*, London: Sage.

Popay, J., Rogers, A. and Williams, G. (1998) 'Rationale and standards for the systematic review of qualitative literature in health services research', *Qualitative Health Research*, 8: 341–51.

Roberts, E. and Mays, N. (1998) 'Can primary care and community-based models of emergency care substitute for the hospital accident and emergency (A&E) department?', *Health Policy*, 44: 191–214.

Robinson, R. (2000) 'Managed care in the United States: a dilemma for evidence-based policy?', *Health Economics*, 9: 1–7.

Robinson, R. and Steiner, A. (1998) *Managed Health Care: US Evidence and Lessons for the National Health Service*, Buckingham: Open University Press.

Sheldon, T. (2001) 'It ain't what you do but the way that you do it', *Journal of Health Services Research and Policy*, 6: 3–5

Steiner, A. and Robinson, R. (1998) 'Managed care: US research evidence and its lessons for the NHS', *Journal of Health Services Research and Policy*, 3: 173–84.

Ukoumunne, O. C., Gulliford, M. C., Chinn, S., Sterne, J. A. C., Burney, P. G. J. and Donner, A. (1999) 'Evaluation of health interventions at area and organisational level', *British Medical Journal*, 319: 376–9.

Williams, F., Popay, J. and Oakley, A. (1999) *Welfare Research: A Critical Review*, London: UCL Press.

Wood, J. and Freemantle, N. (1999) 'Choosing an appropriate unit of analysis in trials of interventions that attempt to influence practice', *Journal of Health Services Research and Policy*, 4: 44–8.

Index